ROMY DOLLÉ

GOOD FAT
BAD FAT

Library of Congress Control Number: 2016932160
Library of Congress Cataloging-in-Publication Data is on file with the publisher
Romy Dollé 1970-
Good Fat, Bad Fat/Romy Dollé

ISBN: 978-1-939563-27-9
1. Health 2. Weight Loss 3. Diet 4. Physical Fitness

Ideas and Recipes: Romy Dollé www.romydolle.com www.davedolle.com
Food staging and photography: Upper Grade AG, 8038 Zurich www.uppergrade.com
Layout and typesetting: Upper Grade AG and Caroline De Vita
Cover Design: Janée Meadows

Publisher: Primal Blueprint Publishing, 1641 S. Rose Ave., Oxnard, CA 93033
For information on quantity discounts, please call 888-774-6259,
email: info@primalblueprintpublishing.com,
or visit PrimalBlueprintPublishing.com.

DISCLAIMER: The ideas, concepts, and opinions expressed in this book are intended to be used for educational purposes only. This book is sold with the understanding that the author and publisher are not rendering medical advice of any kind, nor is this book intended to replace medical advice, nor to diagnose, prescribe, or treat any disease, condition, illness, or injury. It is imperative that before beginning any diet, exercise, or lifestyle program, including any aspect of the methodologies mentioned in *Good Fat, Bad Fat*, you receive full medical clearance from a licensed physician. The author and publisher claim no responsibility to any person or entity for any liability, loss, or damage caused or alleged to be caused directly or indirectly as a result of the use, application, or interpretation of the material in this book. If you object to this disclaimer, you may return the book to the publisher for a full refund.

CONTENTS

RECIPE DIRECTORY

Recipe	Pages	Fat Source
Basil Guacamole	56–57	Avocado
Wasabi Guacamole	56–57	Avocado
Mango Guacamole	56–57	Avocado
Avocado Salad Dressing	58–59	Avocado, Olive Oil
Avocado Smoothie	60-61	Avocado
Egg In Avocado	62-63	Avocado, Egg Yolk, Milk Fat
Chocolate Cream	64-65	Avocado, Cocoa Butter
Coconut Cream	70-71	Coconut Oil
Coconut-Banana Smoothie	72–73	Coconut Oil
Coconut-Beet Smoothie	72–73	Coconut Oil
Coconut-Blueberry Smoothie	72–73	Coconut Oil
Coconut Kaiserschmarrn	74–75	Coconut Oil, Egg Yolk
Paleo Curry	76–77	Coconut Oil
Coconut Sweet Potato Chips	78–79	Coconut Oil
Coconut Pudding	80–81	Coconut Oil
Coconut Macaroons	82–83	Coconut Oil
Cinnamon Coconut Ice Cream	84–85	Coconut Oil, Egg Yolk
Spiced Olive Oils	88-89	Olive Oil
Olives In Prosciutto	90-91	Olive Oil, Lard
Green And Black Tapenade	92-93	Olive Oil
Schnitzel Rolls With Tapenade Filling	94-95	Olive Oil, Lard
Parsnip or Parsley Root Puree	96-97	Olive Oil
Sweet Potato or Potato Puree	96-97	Olive Oil
Cauliflower Puree	96-97	Olive Oil
Olive Oil Cake	98-99	Olive Oil, Egg Yolk
Nut Muesli	102-103	Nuts
Muesli With Raw Milk	104-105	Nuts, Milk Fat
Muesli with Coconut Milk	104-105	Nuts, Coconut Oil
Chocolate-Nut Butter	106-107	Nuts, Cocoa Butter
Fish In Nut Crust	108-109	Nuts, Fish Oil
Nut Pesto	110-111	Nuts, Olive Oil , Milk Fat
Asparagus Noodles With Walnut Pesto	110-111	Nuts, Olive Oil
Apple With Nut Filling	112-113	Nuts, Milk Fat, Coconut Oil
Almond-Chocolate Biscotti	114-115	Nuts, Egg Yolk
Fried Bacon With Popovers	120-121	Lard, Egg Yolk
Rice Noodles With Carbonara Sauce	122-123	Lard, Egg Yolks, Olive Oil
Marinated Pork Belly	124-125	Lard
Porks Chop With Asian Salad	126-127	Lard, Milk Fat

Unbreaded Cordon Bleu	128–129	Lard, Milk Fat
Beef Marrow	134–135	Beef Fat
Merguez (North African Sausages)	136–137	Beef Fat
Thai Veal Shanks	138–139	Beef Fat
DIY Beef Tartare	140–141	Beef Fat, Egg Yolk
Liver Saltimbocca With Butternut Squash	142–143	Beef Fat, Lard, Milk Fat
Lamb Chops	146–147	Lamb Fat
Leg Of Lamb With Sweet Potatoes	148–149	Lamb Fat, Olive Oil
Oriental Lamb Stew	150–151	Lamb Fat, Milk Fat
Signature Lamb Burger With Tzatziki	152–153	Lamb Fat , Milk Fat, Lard, Olive Oil
Chicken Soup	156–157	Chicken Fat
Crispy Chicken Wings	158–159	Chicken Fat
Chicken Liver Pâté	160–161	Chicken Fat, Milk Fat
Butterfly Chicken	162–163	Poultry Fat
Duck Breast Or Quail	164–165	Poultry Fat
Sardine Salad	170–171	Fish Oil, Olive Oil
Braised, Baked Fish	172–173	Fish Oil
Fish Tartare	174–175	Fish Oil, Egg Yolk, Avocado
Caesar Salad with Sweet Potato Croutons	176–177	Fish Oil, Egg Yolks, Olive Oil , Fat
Fish And Vegetable Sticks	178–179	Fish Oil, Coconut Oil
Italian Herb Butter	184–185	Milk Fat
Anchovy Butter	184–185	Milk Fat, Fish Oil
Chive Butter	184–185	Milk Fat
Tomato Butter	184–185	Milk Fat
Rösti With Fried Egg	186–187	Milk Fat, Egg Yolks
Butter Chicken	188–189	Milk Fat, Chicken Fat
Chocolate Pavlova With Cocoa Quark Cream	190–191	Milk Fat
Butter Coffee	192–193	Milkfat
Coconut Coffee	192–193	Coconut Oil
Smoothie With Egg	196–197	Egg Yolk, Avocado
Basic Olive Oil Mayonnaise	198–199	Egg Yolks, Olive Oil
Tomato Mayonnaise	198–199	Yolk, Avocado
Herb Mayonnaise	198–199	Egg Yolks, Olive Oil
Wasabi Mayonnaise	198–199	Egg Yolks, Olive Oil
Sweet Potato-Shrimp Salad	200–201	Egg Yolks, Olive Oil
Cheese Omelette	202–203	Yolk, Milk Fat
Eggs And Vegetable Salad	204–205	Egg Yolks, Olive Oil
Chocolate Mousse	206–207	Yolk, Cocoa Butter
Pure Food Chocolate	210–211	Cocoa Butter

INTRO

BEFORE: FAT-FREE QUARK, CHICKEN BREASTS, AND EGG WHITE OMELETTES

For years I ate a strict low-fat diet. I knew how many calories and especially how much fat was in every morsel of food I touched. I didn't want to be fat, and the science (led by Ancel Keys) told me that obesity was highest in countries where people ate the most fat.

That research made sense to me: One gram of fat has nine calories, and a gram of carbohydrates or a gram of protein only four calories. I could eat twice as much food if I just left out the fat!

On my strict low-fat diet, I was certainly slim. But that's about the only benefit I can think of. And I wasn't slim just from eating a low-fat diet—I also had to watch closely my daily calorie intake.

I was hungry almost all the time. I didn't want to eat too much, so I stayed hungry and was often in a terrible mood. I was unbalanced and about as far from a morning person as you can imagine, even after I ate breakfast. I drank coffee until I felt a bit better. I hid behind my computer screen at the office and just wanted to be left alone. Fortunately, I didn't have any interactions with customers in the morning. (Fortunately for the customers, that is.)

Some days my bad mood lasted all day, and I wallowed in it. I'd put on my dark glasses and ignore everyone.

On top of these mental effects, I suffered physically. Although I was slim, I wasn't fit or firm. My belly made me look four months pregnant. I regularly had severe, unpleasant flatulence and chronic constipation. I caught colds all the time, most of which lasted for weeks.

I tried everything to get rid of my belly, but through every diet and miracle cure I tried, I always kept my diet low in fat. I firmly believed that "fat makes you fat."

BUTTER, FRIED BACON, AVOCADO, AND COCONUT

Since I began to fill my diet with fat, nutrient-rich foods, I've become a different person. I almost can't believe the difference in myself. I'm happy and balanced and look forward to getting up every morning. I'm filled with energy and creativity. I enjoy life and eat when I'm hungry.

I'm in better shape than ever, at almost forty-six years old. I have visible abdominal muscles! I love them. I'm muscular and strong. I haven't been sick for years, not even with one of those colds I used to get all the time.

WHAT CHANGED MY MIND ABOUT FAT?

Through my research on healthy eating and the scrupulous testing of a wide variety of diets, I came across the Paleo diet. The Paleo approach is unjustly characterized as simply a meat-heavy diet. In fact, it's a perfectly balanced way of eating, advocating a diet made up of 30 percent proteins, 30 percent carbohydrates, and 40 percent fat. Eating Paleo means eliminating all grains, freeing up carbohydrate calories, which are replaced by fat (because calorie restriction is not part of Paleo eating).

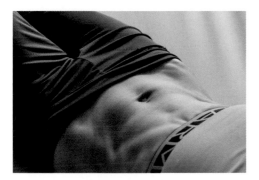

Yes, I have dared to include healthy fats and oils in my diet. And adding fat hasn't just made me healthy—it's made food taste better, and eating has become fun and enjoyable. I immediately became more relaxed around food and eating, and I started to discover and love new dishes and foods. After a while, eating wasn't just about about getting nutrients into my body

anymore; it became instead a journey of discovery through the universe of flavor and aroma. I ate fatty cuts of meat, like lamb chops, with vegetables slathered in butter. I had crispy organic bacon at Sunday brunch—a pleasure I had denied myself for years. One of my favorite new meals, both in taste and because it's a veritable nutrient bomb, is roasted beef marrow, which we eat directly from the bone with a spoon or serve over grilled vegetables.

Of course, there is still a lot to discover on my journey to ultimate health and being a gourmandise. The nice thing about this journey is that it perfectly harmonizes both goals—being healthy and revelling in the pleasure of food.

EVOLUTION

Nutrition science is changing—and it will continue to change. As we learn, we must keep re-interpreting what we thought we knew. To understand which food makes us thrive and why, we need to understand the evolution of humanity and how food affects our brain. So I hope you'll come with me as we explore the history of the Stone Age people.

Our ancestors from the Paleolithic era hunted to satisfy the basic need of hunger. These hunter-gatherers ate a more balanced diet than we previously assumed. They didn't eat any grains or dairy products but ate many species of plants, nuts, and mushrooms, as well as meat. According to the evolutionary biologist Ulrich Kutschera, our Paleolithic ancestors ate a lot of fat. From 40 to 50 percent of their diet consisted of wild animal meat, supplemented with nuts, berries, fruits, and vegetables. Because food storage options were very limited, and food had to be found every day, anyone who did not hunt or gather starved. Our ancestors were constantly seeking food, meaning they were constantly in motion. The diet of the hunter-gatherers shows that a lower-carb, high-fat diet can support levels of physical activity virtually unknown in the modern world.

People's eating habits changed fundamentally with the advent of agriculture about ten thousand years ago. On the menu were more carbohydrates and less protein and fat. Kutschera's opinion is that this modified diet is at the root of many of today's most widespread diseases, such as cancer, diabetes, and obesity.

CEREAL CROPS COULD BE STORED—PEOPLE NO LONGER NEED TO FIND FOOD EVERY DAY.

Lucrative income from farming attracted people, and villages developed. As people came together, conversations arose, out of which emerged new, creative ideas. Technological progress supported the rapid development of new products that were exchanged and traded—trade bloomed.

So the development of agriculture was a milestone in the history of humanity and changed life as we know it. The height of the trade and agriculture economy in Europe was reached during the Roman Empire: orchards, vegetable gardens, and cornfields were farmed. The nobility enjoyed rich feasts and had meals that flaunted their status. But commoners often suffered from famine and ate little more than bread, vegetables, cereals, and legumes.

In the nineteenth century, industrialization became more important than agriculture in many places; thus, the era of the food industry began. Convenience foods eventually became popular—products like powdered mashed potatoes, which were prepared just by mixing the powder with hot water.

The agricultural habits of people changed fundamentally ten thousand years ago.

THE CHANGE
FAT PHOBIA AND
LOW-FAT PRODUCTS

With the invention of agriculture, the high-fat diet shifted to a carbohydrate-rich diet—and the number of obese people increased every year. The view that excessive consumption of carbohydrates and sweets was the cause of obesity was replaced in the seventies and eighties by the assumption that fat was the culprit, and the low-fat movement flourished. In the National Nutrition Survey of 1991, participants said that vegetables, fruit, and salad were the most important foods for a balanced diet, followed by milk, cottage cheese/yogurt, bread, and potatoes. Fat was classified as moderately unhealthy, though healthier than sweets, and after the sweets came fatty meat, sugar, beer, and alcohol.

Although foods with a super low fat percentage were being manufactured and marketed aggressively, people were getting fatter. According to the German Society for Nutrition, the incidence of overweight people (both pre-obese and obese) poses one of the greatest challenges for health care in the twenty-first century. Being overweight is a risk factor for diabetes, hypertension, metabolic disease, cardiovascular disorders, and psychological problems. And experts now believe that it's actually carbohydrates from sugary and starchy foods making people fatter.

OUR SENSES GET OVERWHELMED BY THE WIDE RANGE OF CONSUMER GOODS AVAILABLE.

The huge supply in grocery stores dictates what people purchase, and the advertising industry creates our "needs." We're manipulated in the supermarket and influenced by marketing. Every day we are exposed to an enormous number of stimuli; according to Ingrid Kiefer and Cem Ekmekcioglu, we have to make about two hundred food-related decisions in the course of a single day. Gorgeous models influence our decision-making, as does the wide variety in the supermarket, and our emotions are triggered.

Every society since time immemorial has upheld an ideal of female beauty. But each epoch has seen the ideal differently: In the Middle Ages, pale skin was a great marker of beauty. Later, rounder and more curvaceous women became the ideal—we refer to these women as "Rubenesque" after the baroque painter Peter Paul Rubens, who famously painted voluptuous women. This ideal was adjusted again with the introduction of the corset to create artificially tiny waists; then, in the twentieth century, corsets were phased out.

Though a chubby physique once signified wealth, today the opposite is true—we think of skinniness as elegant and wealthy people as mostly slim.

Food for folks in the Stone Age was a matter of sheer survival; in the twentieth century, we became inundated by fast-food chains, pizza delivery services, and restaurants. We felt entitled to acquire as much as possible with as little effort as possible, and we were happy with every new fast-food joint that opened, ignoring the evidence that our diet was slowly leading to an alarming rise in obesity.

In the fifties there was a huge increase in cardiovascular diseases—a rude awakening for a nation becoming addicted to convenience foods.

There were two main scientists working to solve the puzzle of why people were becoming fatter and experiencing a crisis of cardiovascular disease. Ancel Keys believed the culprits were saturated fat and high cholesterol; John Yudkin recognized the dangers of excessive consumption of sugar. Keys, by far the more politically astute of the two, won the public over, and fat phobia began.

Today, we are better understanding how Keys's research was deeply flawed. His famous "seven-country study" certainly confirmed his theory that dietary fat, particularly saturated fat, was contributing to obesity and heart disease. But he neglected to include studies of five other countries that proved the absolute contrary in his final report. Unfortunately, there was not enough scrutiny of his techniques at the time, and the hysteria around cholesterol began. At a much later date, Ancel Keys admitted there was no relationship between dietary cholesterol and blood cholesterol, but that hasn't made a dent in our collective panic about cholesterol and fat consumption. Grocery stores reinforce the hysteria, crammed with "lite" products like skim milk and low-fat chips. The theory that we need to eat fat for our bodies to function optimally seems, to most people, outrageous. To make the public aware that natural fat is healthy, we need much more scientific evidence disseminated among the general population.

DR. TORSTEN ALBERS
CHOLESTEROL AND CHOLESTEROL METABOLISM

There are three types of lipoproteins (fat-protein particles): VLDL (very low density lipoprotein), LDL (low density lipoprotein), and HDL (high density lipoprotein). In all three types, there are particles that contain a mixture of triglycerides, cholesterol, and phospholipids. VLDL is particularly high in triglycerides, LDL contains a lower amount of fat molecules, and HDL is low in triglycerides but rich in protein.

The harmfulness of lipoproteins is assessed differently. VLDL and LDL are considered "bad" for arteries, and increased levels of these are a risk factor for vascular infarction and premature cardiac death. HDL, on the other hand, is regarded as a protective factor against coronary heart disease—it is considered more likely to protect blood vessels. This is because of, among other things, the fact that VLDL and LDL transport cholesterol *away from* the liver to supply the cells of the body, while HDL transports cholesterol back to the liver, where it is recycled and reused. So if you have high LDL and low HDL levels, this means you have an increased risk factor for the biggest killer in the western world: heart attack. If your LDL levels are within the normal range and your HDL levels are increased, your total cholesterol may well be significantly higher than normal, but this doesn't mean you have to worry.

Conversely, however, your total cholesterol can still be in the normal range, but if you have low HDL and high LDL values, you'll still show an increased risk for early heart attack. Thus, the total cholesterol level in the blood is not a good parameter for assessing the risk factor of lipid metabolism disorders. Rather, we must take a different approach in order to make a reasonable assessment.

Official recommended reference values of the different lipoproteins and triglycerides in the blood

Lipoprotein	Standard Value (mmol / l)	Standard Value (mg/dl)	Notes
Total Cholesterol	<5	<200	
LDL	<4	<160	No or only one risk factor for vascular disease (such as smoking, high blood pressure, stress, obesity, etc.)
	<2.5	<100	Two or more risk factors for vascular disease
	<1.75	<70	With preexisting heart disease or diagnosed diabetes
HDL	>1.0 (men)	>40	
	>1.2 (women)	>50	
Triglycerides	< 1.70	<150	

There are rare, congenital lipoprotein disorders where the LDL and total cholesterol are extremely high (>10 mmol/l or >12 mmol/l). Affected patients often get their first heart attack before the age of thirty. Such patients have to take high dosages of lipid-lowering drugs to minimize the risk of early heart attack. In most cases, however, people with elevated cholesterol and LDL levels have good success with consistent lifestyle changes: giving up smoking, getting regular physical activity, reducing weight and body fat,

and changing dietary habits. In my experience, patients making these lifestyle changes can expect a decrease in cholesterol levels of 20 to 40 percent. Often a lifelong drug therapy isn't necessary when lifestyle changes are implemented permanently.

Cholesterol intake through food affects blood cholesterol by only 10 to 15 percent. Reducing daily intake of eggs and high-fat animal foods doesn't actually affect the blood lipid levels significantly.

LETTING FAT OFF THE HOOK

Gary Taubes, a science writer and the author of *Why We Get Fat* and *Good Calories, Bad Calories*, is of the opinion that you don't get fat because you eat more; you eat more because you are fat. According to Taubes, the metabolism of many people is disturbed because their carbohydrate intake is too high. Eating too many carbohydrates allows the blood sugar levels to rise, which causes a spike in insulin production, which lowers blood sugar levels again. The body burns a certain amount of sugar you consume, but not all the sugar, if it's consumed excessively. What happens to the rest? It's converted into fat and stored in adipose tissue. If the body's cells are insulin resistant, the sugar is not converted to energy and instead becomes fat. If you try to solve the problem of extra body fat with the consumption of low-fat products, it's likely your weight will continue to rise, according to Taubes. He believes that excessive consumption of concentrated carbohydrates leads to lifestyle diseases such as obesity, diabetes, cancer, and Alzheimer's. And Taubes does not believe that increased fat consumption results in unfavorable cholesterol levels or cardiovascular disease.

The book *Krebszellen lieben Zucker — Patienten brauchen Fett* (in English, *Cancer Cells Love Sugar — Patients Need Fat*) by Ulrike Kämmerer, Dr. Schlatterer and Dr. Knoll, details how and why a fat-rich diet (especially omega-3 fatty acids) may be useful in fighting cancer and other diseases—that fat can be good medicine rather than the poison we've been led to believe. Ulrike Kämmerer was one of the researchers of Universitätsfrauenklinik Würzburg (a university hospital in Würzburg, Germany) who carried out a study with sixteen cancer patients to see if a high-fat diet would help to make the patients feel better. After three months, patients who were still in the study had an improved quality of life. As a side effect (in this study, not necessarily a desirable one), the cancer patients lost some weight—less than the amount lost with more balanced diets.

The study by Jay Wortman is also interesting. According to Wortman, the residents of a small Canadian village where mostly fishers live have one thing in common: they love calorie-dense food. Residents there eat pizza, fries, ice cream, and burgers daily. The consequences? They suffer from rates of diabetes, cardiovascular disease, and metabolic syndromes five times higher than the average Canadian. After seeing the eating habits and health problems of these people, Wortman suggested to them that they implement an Atkins diet. The eighty-six obese people there began eating their burgers without buns, more salmon, bacon, eggs, and vegetables. Despite their increased consumption of fat, the people became leaner. One year later, most of them had lost 26 pounds or more. But Wortman was even more interested in the positive change in blood markers than the weight loss. With the low-carb, high-fat diet, triglycerides were optimized and the blood glucose levels were down, vastly improving health. Many in the community on the diet were able to stop taking their medication for diabetes.

Yudkin's theory that sugar is the culprit, not fat, is also gaining popularity. Dr. Robert Lustig, an American scientist and author, suggests the same idea with his 2009 lecture "Sugar: The Bitter Truth." Robert Atkins's book *Dr. Atkins' Diet Revolution* (1972) also emphasized that eating high-fat foods such as steaks, eggs, and butter would lead to weight loss, and that pasta, rice, bagels, and sugar were mainly responsible for Western obesity. Atkins's book sold millions of copies.

OUR MIND AFFECTS OUR EATING HABITS

What we eat can have a positive as well as a negative effect on our bodies and our behavior. Our food memories and associations are a huge factor in whether or not we like to eat certain foods. Most of us have a strong emotional attachment to meals from our childhood, for example, and eating them is comforting.

Eating something delicious is especially gratifying to our emotions—it's a delight to our palate. Delicious foods tend to contain fat—fat amplifies flavor and also satiety. If your main course is delicious (and deliciously fatty), you'll have less desire to eat more food afterwards. Someone who eats tasteless food—for example, low-fat cheese—runs the risk of not feeling sated. Food with a bit of sugar and a lot of fat is very appealing to our palates. If the fat content is reduced, the flavor and deliciousness of a food is reduced as well. And yet, because the satiety fat provides is missing, we get cravings for more of those not-so-delicious foods. It's even believed that a lower fat intake introduces emotions such as fear and hostility. With increased fat intake, on the other hand, anxiety and tension decrease. To understand why we follow certain patterns of behavior and why we give up certain foods and prefer others, we need to understand what's happening in our brain when we eat.

HOW DOES OUR BRAIN WORK?

Today we can divide food into roughly two types: natural and industrially produced. Many industrially produced foods trigger the release of dopamine, which means that if you eat them regularly, they become addictive. Scientists call the brain getting used to something "neuroadaptation." Nerve cells transmit a subjective reality to the brain.

Lisle and Goldhamer, in their book *The Pleasure Trap*, provide a good analogy to understand this concept: Imagine we are in a dark room. Suddenly the light is switched on. We feel dazzled briefly until the message "It is now brighter" reaches the brain. Now the brain can tell our pupils to become smaller, and our visual sensitivity is optimized.

Now let's go outside, where the sun is shining, and allow our eyes to adjust to the bright sunlight. Good! When we return to the room once more, the light seems rather dim, even though just a minute ago it seemed too bright. As Lisle and Goldhamer say, "Our perception is therefore a response to changes in relative but not absolute stimulation grade." This example shows how we adapt to almost any sensory input. In the same way, we have become accustomed over time to new flavors: we've become so used to industrially and chemically manufactured foods that we want salt and sugar in all of our food. Food without salt and/or sugar added seems tasteless and bland. To wean ourselves from the flavors we're used to is not a simple endeavor. (And does any of this sound familiar—like after-school specials warning you about drug addictions? That's because drugs work the same way. Take a drug regularly and your body gets used to it and wants more and more.)

HUNGER AND SATIETY

Every person comes with a healthy sense of satiety. The mechanism of hunger and satiety is a complex process controlled by the central nervous system. There are messengers that signal satiety and others that stimulate hunger. And we need to distinguish hunger from appetite: according to Kiefer and Ekmekcioglu, hunger is an uncomfortable, painful craving for food, and appetite is a more lustful motivation.

Hunger does not originate in the stomach. Your stomach growling is not a hunger signal—it's just the walls of your stomach contracting. Hunger signals come from blood sugar levels; a low blood sugar level sends signals via receptors in the liver and stomach to the hypothalamus, where the control system for the autonomic nervous system resides. So then, why do we feel full? Because food expands the stomach. The nerves in the stomach send that information to the hypothalamus and other parts of the brain, which produce a feeling of satiety.

The hormones in the body are also responsible for hunger and satiety signals. The hormone ghrelin, which is generated in the stomach, intestines, hypothalamus, and the pituitary gland, signals hunger; the hormone leptin signals satiety. Lack of sleep can suppress leptin, which means we tend to be hungrier when we haven't slept well.

APPETITE, HUNGER AND CRAVINGS

Appetite is more of a mental phenomenon, not always related to hunger. We can have an appetite for a food, even if we are not hungry. Ravenous hunger often occurs for hormonal reasons (pregnancy or the menstrual cycle). Cravings may even be accompanied by shivering and sweating. Usually this kind of appetite is centered around sweets. The serotonin increase after we eat sugar does spike our happiness—but it's temporary! Soon afterward, the body wants more of the happy-making substance, in this case sugar. The whole process of ingestion is a complex interaction of various processes in the brain, stomach, and intestines.

EMOTIONAL EATING

Emotions have a significant impact on our eating habits. If we experience positive or negative feelings while we're eating, we call it "emotional eating." As early as infancy, we learn that if we cry, we'll be soothed with food. Later, toddlers and older children are told that if they eat just a few more bites, they'll be given dessert. This kind of coerced feeding and the sweet reward at the end disturbs the child's instinctive ability to recognize satiety. The child's subconscious begins to intrinsically link emotions, ambience, the availability of food, being with other people, smells, and other habits with their eating behavior, and emotional eating is cemented.

"Decisions are made with awareness—habits are not." Thanks to Ivan Petrovich Pavlov's experiments with his famous "Pavlovian dogs," we know that at the sight or smell of food, saliva production increases. Pavlov's dogs began salivating when they heard Pavlov's footsteps, without having any food in front of them. Pavlov's behavioral learning theory is that if the dog can react with more saliva while listening to the steps of its owner, another trigger could be used, such as a ringing bell.

Using the same principles, we can reverse our emotional eating habits. Habits, such as the timing of our meals, are very important in our daily lives—they give us stability. If we change a habit such as mealtime, or are forced to change it, this leads to turmoil and stress.

Food can regulate emotions, anxiety, and stress, make us happy, and even replace love. Because food distracts us from our feelings, we tend to overeat when we're dealing with negative feelings. Also, anger and argumentativeness are linked to a low-fat, high-sugar diet, and on stressful days we tend to eat high-fat, high-sugar foods.

If our negative emotional eating habits become pathological, they are called bulimia, anorexia nervosa, or binge eating. Binge eaters don't necessarily have a problem with their weight as do people suffering from anorexia or bulimia. Binge eaters have episodes of overeating due to mental stress. Everybody knows the feeling of sitting down after a stressful day with some comfort food. You have seconds at dinner, and some ice cream while you're watching TV—you've earned it! Feelings and negative emotions make it difficult to understand how much food we actually need. Rather than searching for the true reason for our cravings, we try to suppress them with food.

Maybe it's not surprising that the diseases of civilization of the twenty-first century include obesity, diabetes, and cardiovascular disease.

DR. TORSTEN ALBERS
THE COMPLICATIONS OF BEING OVERWEIGHT OR OBESE

While it was previously thought that fat was merely a passive storage tissue, today it's known that fat cells are very metabolically active. They secrete different substances and signaling molecules called adipokines. These are secreted more when there is an increase in fat cell size. These signaling substances affect:

- Blood pressure
- Inflammatory process
- Insulin and glucose metabolism
- Blood clotting

So being overweight or obese means, for example, an increase in blood pressure because of the increase in adipokines being secreted from enlarged fat cells. Simultaneously, these adipokines will also accelerate vascular aging, increase insulin and glucose levels in the blood, and will increase the risk of blood clot formation in the vessels (e.g., in the context of a thrombosis). Conversely, if someone experiences a partial "emptying" of fat cells as part of a weight loss, the effects will be the opposite, and thus positive on these parameters, which is attributable to the declining secretion of adipokines from the smaller fat cells. Thus, decreased fat cell size = low secretion of adipokines = good for health. Increased fat cell size = high secretion of adipokines = bad for health.

Beyond these mechanisms of the altered release of adipokines by fat cells, the risk of developing these diseases increases drastically with obesity, meaning increased fat mass:

- Type II diabetes
- Arterial hypertension
- Dyslipidemia: low HDL cholesterol (or "good" cholesterol), elevated LDL cholesterol (or "bad" cholesterol), high triglycerides (fats flooding the blood)
- Metabolic syndrome (chronically elevated insulin levels are linked to the common occurrence of obesity, high blood pressure, increased "bad" cholesterol, and impaired glucose tolerance, or pre-diabetes)
- Accelerated atherosclerosis ("hardening of the arteries") with premature heart attack/stroke
- Different types of cancer (especially breast cancer, colon cancer)
- Depression

- Back pain
- Osteoarthritis ("wear" of the cartilage)
- Non-alcoholic fatty liver disease progressing to inflammation of the liver and cirrhosis, as well as leading to chronic renal failure and premature heart attack
- Osteoporosis (loss of bone mass with increased risk of fractures and pain)
- Sleep apnea (multiple cessation of breathing during sleep with resulting daytime sleepiness)

Of course, these diseases and conditions don't automatically occur in every obese person. However, the likelihood of developing them increases with body fat, to sometimes more than ten times! Even obese children are at risk, developing what we used to call "adult onset" diabetes (because people didn't develop it until they were forty or fifty years old) at age fourteen or fifteen.

FAT FACTS
WHY DO WE NEED FAT?

Fat:
- Supplies energy
- Carries fat-soluble vitamins A, D, E, and K
- Acts as an important flavor carrier
- Is a building material for cells of all types (nerve, brain, and immune cells)
- Supplies essential fatty acids, which the body cannot generate itself
- Stores energy (fat deposits)
- Provides impact and pressure protection for the organs in the body
- Is a thermoregulator

Every cell in our body needs fat to function. Fat is the building material for nerve, brain, and immune cells, and it's important for balanced hormone production. In addition, it helps to create beautiful skin and healthy hair, and it regulates digestion. It carries the fat-soluble vitamin substances A, D, E, and K, and it's an important flavor carrier.

Fat deposits also provide shock and pressure protection for our bodies. Fat keeps us warm and stores energy well.

Carbohydrates are not essential; a person can be healthy, strong, and long-lived without them. In parts of the world, Stone Age humans lived with very few carbohydrates and were in excellent physical condition. Their notorious low life expectancy was mainly due to hunting accidents and infectious diseases. They suffered, in contrast to today, hardly any degenerative or chronic diseases such as heart attacks, stroke, or cancer.

Fat is the healthiest fuel for our body, and it provides more than twice as much energy as the same amount of carbohydrates and protein.

Especially valuable as an energy source is fat that includes many natural nutrients. These nutrients are found in abundance in:

- Organic pastured beef
- Organic pastured veal
- Organic pastured pork
- Organic pastured lamb
- Wild game (deer, moose, wild boar, etc.)
- Organic fatty fish
- Free-range chicken
- Egg yolks from free-range chickens
- Organic clarified butter or ghee from grass-fed cows
- Organic avocado
- Extra-virgin coconut and palm oil
- Cold-pressed extra-virgin olive oil
- Organic nuts, raw or dry roasted

These fats contain all the essential fatty acids that cannot be produced by the human body.

The animal products, however, only contain sufficient fatty acids if the animals were fed well and humanely raised. Cattle should, for example, only eat pasture grass and hay. Calves should only drink the milk of pasture-fed cows. Animals pastured and treated well don't fall ill as much and won't need antibiotics to stay healthy.

The same applies to all the other animals. They must live and eat the way they would in the wild. Chickens would walk around all day in the open air and eat insects, worms, larvae and snails, and from time to time a seed or grain. They would certainly not feed mainly on grains. But what do industrially farmed chickens eat today? Grains and soy. Some growers boast that they feed their animals organic grains and sell their "organic eggs"— but these animals and their eggs contain none of the healthy natural fatty acids, because they're not being fed naturally.

Incidentally, this also applies to farmed fish, which aren't fed with animal-friendly, biologically problem-free nutrients.

Butter and clarified butter (also called ghee; I'll use these terms interchangeably) can only contain healthy fatty acids if the cow is pastured, does not receive antibiotics, and isn't stressed by an unnatural, caged habitat (i.e., a narrow livestock stall).

In the case of coconut oil, palm oil, and olive oil, it is extremely important that these have not been processed industrially. Through the industrial manufacturing process, natural healthy fatty acids are destroyed, making unhealthy trans fats instead.

DR. TORSTEN ALBERS
FAT DIGESTION AND METABOLISM

Fats (chemically speaking, triglycerides) are digested by fat-digesting enzymes in the stomach (15 percent) and by special lipases from the pancreas in the duodenum (85 percent)—producing free fatty acids. Monoacylglycerines (glycerol with one fatty acid molecule, unlike triglycerides, which are glycerol with three fatty acid molecules) are absorbed from the cells of the intestines and re-esterified to complete triglycerides. Then these triglycerides are submitted (along with cholesterol and phospholipids) to the lymphatic system in the form of chylomicrons. These chylomicrons transport lipids to the muscle cells, cardiac cells, and fat cells, and some eventually reach the liver.

In fat cells the fatty acids get re-esterified and stored as triglycerides. Muscle cells can burn triglycerides directly. One to two hours after a carbohydrate- and fat-rich meal (e.g., spaghetti Bolognese, cheese pizza, high-fat sweets), many chylomicrons appear in the blood, and a large proportion of triglycerides are absorbed by fat cells. Since the carbohydrates of a meal are the primary fuel for muscles, after such a meal only glucose oxidation occurs, while most of the ingested fat is stored.

HOW DOES THE BODY GENERATE ENERGY?

Our body can create energy two ways. It can burn fatty acids, in a process called fat oxidation. It can also burn carbohydrates, or sugar, in a process called glucose oxidation. Which method your body uses depends on the proportion of carbohydrates to fat in your diet. As long as you regularly eat a lot of carbs (especially sugar and grains), your body will be burning those carbs for energy, and it won't burn fat. This means our bodies have basically "unlearned" how to extract energy from fat, because we've been consuming so many carbs.

Because our capacity to store glucose is small compared to our capacity for fat storage, if we're burning sugar for energy, our body demands frequent replenishment. Ever felt like you can't think clearly and crave sweets? Shortly after you eat the sugar, you feel better, more relaxed, and your head is clear once more.

But those sweet foods only fill your energy needs (and psychological ones) temporarily. Over the long term, you're in a terrible cycle. When you consume sugar, your blood glucose level rises. This stimulates your pancreas to produce insulin. The insulin enters the bloodstream and moves the sugar from your blood into your cells—causing your blood sugar levels to take a nosedive. This rapid rise in blood sugar levels, followed by high insulin production and then an abrupt slump, leaves you feeling hungry again, even though you've consumed enough calories. All the extra calories you end up eating are stored in body fat deposits.

In a low-carbohydrate, high-fat diet, the capacity for burning fat for energy in your muscle cells increases. If you eat less than 1 to 1.7 oz (30 to 50 g) of carbohydrates per day, your body produces ketone bodies (this is called ketogenesis).

The brain can use these ketone bodies for fuel instead of glucose. That makes the brain independent from carbohydrates in your food. This is an automatic process which our ancestors' bodies developed in periods of famine. Human bodies can not only get energy from fat but can thrive—physically and mentally—without carbohydrates. This is important not only for overweight people but also for all health-conscious people; a low-carbohydrate diet and more stable blood sugar levels reduce the risk of developing diabetes and many other diseases.

HOW CAN I ACTIVATE FAT METABOLISM?

- Avoid sugar
- Avoid simple carbohydrates
- In general, eat few carbohydrates
- Eat more short and medium fats and oils (I'll explain these)
- Don't snack

WHAT IS A KETOGENIC DIET?

In a ketogenic diet, the daily carbohydrate intake is less than 1 to 1.7 oz (30 to 50 g). The diet consists of only meat, fish, eggs, cheese, cream, non-starchy vegetables, nuts, and seeds, supplemented with butter, coconut oil, mayonnaise, and other healthy fats. The fat intake is much higher than in a standard diet and provides about 75 to 85 percent of the total calories. Protein then provides the remaining calories. This diet became well known in the latter half of the twentieth century as the Atkins diet, named after American physician Dr. Robert Atkins.

In this diet, blood sugar levels don't spike, so the insulin level decreases greatly and the release of fatty acids from adipose tissue and their combustion are in full swing. Here arise so-called "activated acetic acid residues," from which, in turn, arise the ketone bodies. The brain uses ketones as "substitute carbs" to cover up to 75 percent of its energy needs. So it's simply not true that the brain uses exclusively glucose as fuel; however, there will only be appreciable ketone bodies, when, as shown above, very few carbohydrates and a lot of fat are consumed, for at least 36 to 48 hours. With a ketogenic diet you are able to mimic the metabolic status of fasting without the danger of losing muscle mass.

Ketone bodies have a strong hunger-supressing effect. This, together with the additional strong water loss during the first days of this diet, adds up to a lot of weight lost very quickly. As soon as carbohydrate intake rises again, however, body weight increases quickly.

FAT OR OIL?

Depending on whether a fat is liquid or solid at room temperature, it is classified as oil or fat. Butter is for example a fat; it is not liquid at room temperature. The fat of the coconut, however, is liquid at room temperature, and is therefore classified as an oil.

PRODUCTION OF FATS AND OILS

THE GOOD ONES
*   Animal fats are either taken directly from the fatty tissues of animals (pigs, cattle, veal, lamb, poultry, etc.) or melted from milk (butter) obtained by centrifugation.
*   Vegetable fats and oils must be prepared by pressing or extraction. The pressure is a purely mechanical process.

THE BAD ONES
*   Seed and plant oils that need to be heated to high temperatures, then pressed and finally chemically deodorized so they don't taste bad.
*   Chemically produced fats (trans fats) are artificial fatty acids that occur in industrial oil hardening of plant/seed oils. To make these hardened oils palatable, acidifier is added (lactic acid casein, citric acid, whey or yogurt cultures). The yellow color is created by the addition of beta-carotene. Often vitamins A, D, and E are added, as all natural vitamins are destroyed in the manufacturing process.

COMPOSITION OF FATS AND OILS

Fat is composed of various fatty acids, which all have different structures. Each fatty acid has a different role in nutrition and metabolism. We distinguish between:

- Saturated fatty acids
- Monounsaturated fatty acids
- Polyunsaturated fatty acids

A further distinction can be made between essential and non-essential fatty acids. The human body cannot produce essential fatty acids itself, so we must obtain these from our food.

For humans, isoleucine, histidine, leucine, lysine, methionine, phenylalanine, threonine, tryptophan, and valine are considered vital amino acids. Arginine is considered vital only in certain situations, such as during adolescence or during healing from sickness, an accident, surgery, etc., so is therefore referred to as semi-essential.

Most animal fats and oils are composed mainly of saturated and to a lesser extent unsaturated fatty acids. There are a few vegetable fats and oils that contain many saturated fatty acids—for example, coconut oil and palm oil (see chart on p. 27). There is no fat or oil that consists only of saturated or unsaturated fatty acids.

FATTY ACID COMPOSITION

Triglycerides are a compound of three fatty acid molecules bound together by a glycerol molecule. They are considered the storage form of fat in the fat cells. Triglycerides are too large to exit the membrane that surrounds the fat cells. In order for them to be released from storage and deposited into the bloodstream for use as energy, triglycerides must be broken down into their component molecules, in other words, "freed" from triglyceride into free fatty acids.

Fatty acids in turn consist of different long chains of carbon atoms. Each fatty acid has its own name, depending on the length of these chains. There are chemical bonds between the carbon atoms—single bonds and double bonds. Depending on the number of bonds a fatty acid contains, it is categorized as saturated or unsaturated (monounsaturated or polyunsaturated).

With saturated fats, all potential bonding sites on the carbon atoms of the fatty acid chain are occupied by hydrogen; hence the term "saturated." Monounsaturated fats contain a single double bond ("mono") in their fatty acid chain. Polyunsaturated fats contain more than one double bond in their fatty acid chain. The more double bonds a fatty acid contains, the more fluid it is. Hence, polyunsaturated oils retain their liquid form at room temperature and even when refrigerated.

AVERAGE FATTY ACID COMPOSITION OF EDIBLE FATS (PERCENTAGE)

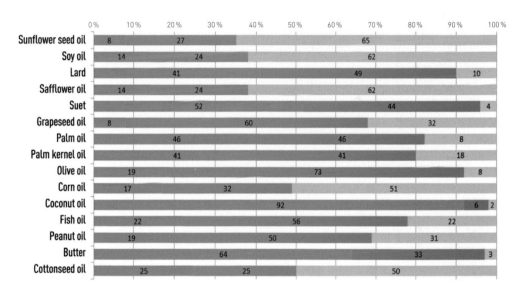

● SATURATED FATTY ACIDS
● MONOUNSATURATED FATTY ACIDS
● POLYUNSATURATED FATTY ACIDS

SATURATED FAT

Saturated fats have the great advantage of being able to withstand high temperatures without becoming unstable. Saturated fatty acids oxidize (i.e., become rancid if they come into contact with oxygen) less rapidly than unsaturated fats. Simply put, they are more durable. Saturated fatty acids are an ideal fuel.

SFA, MUFA, AND PUFA

In saturated fat, no multiple bonds occur. All carbon atoms are fully occupied with hydrogen atoms. Abbreviation: SFA, for saturated fatty acids.

For monounsaturated fatty acids, there is a double bond at one point. One of the most famous sources of monounsaturated fat is olive oil. Avocados also contain these fatty acids. Abbreviation: MUFA, for monounsaturated fatty acids.

Polyunsaturated fatty acids are composed of several double bonds. Most vegetable oils are composed of polyunsaturated fatty acids, and fatty fish contain this fat. The much-vaunted omega-3 and omega-6 fatty acids are also included in this group. Abbreviation: PUFA, for polyunsaturated fatty acids.

The stability of saturated fatty acids is obtained by the joining of carbon atoms. Depending on how many atoms are together, we speak of long chain fatty acids (more than twelve carbon atoms in a row), short chain fatty acids (a maximum of six atoms), and medium chain fatty acids (eight to twelve atoms).

The more hydrogen atoms attached to the carbon atom chain, the more saturated (more stable) the fatty acid.

MONOUNSATURATED FATTY ACIDS

Foods with a high content of monounsaturated fatty acids are likewise quite stable when stored properly and not heated above 350°F (180°C). The body can create monounsaturated fatty acids itself.

POLYUNSATURATES

These fatty acids are the least stable and oxidize very quickly when they come into contact with oxygen. Polyunsaturated fatty acids cannot be manufactured by the body. The known fatty acids omega-6 and omega-3 belong to this group. With these fatty acids, it's not the total amount ingested that's vital to health, but the balance of the two.

THE FATTY ACID RATIO OF OMEGA-6 TO OMEGA-3

Both omega-6 and omega-3 fatty acids are essential. The natural, healthy omega-6 to omega-3 ratio is 1:1 or 2:1. But because of our high consumption of industrially produced vegetable fats and oils (sunflower oil, peanut oil, rapeseed oil, linseed oil, etc.), the ratio in the average citizen is about 20:1. This imbalance is making us sick.

TRANS FATS

Plant fats and oils usually contain many simple and polyunsaturated fatty acids. These are already liquid at low temperatures, go rancid quickly, and cannot withstand high heat. They can't be used by the food industry and they aren't spreadable. Unsaturated fatty acids are treated so that they are "saturated" industrially. Artificially saturated fats (better known as trans fats) are then used for many convenience foods. Trans fats are known to make us insidiously ill for quite some time, often unnoticed at first. They can damage DNA in our cells, weaken our immune system, cause cancer, heart disease, obesity, learning disorders, digestive problems, and much more.

However, we can bring our ratio of omega-6 and omega-3 fatty acids back to ideal by eating the right fats and oils. The most effective way is to reduce consumption of omega-6 fatty acids and increase saturated and polyunsaturated omega-3 fatty acids, so choose:

- Organic butter instead of margarine
- Clarified butter or ghee for frying instead of vegetable fats or oil
- Organic coconut oil for frying
- Fatty organic meat instead of lean meat
- Organic oily fish instead of lean fish
- Avocado
- Cold-pressed extra-virgin olive oil (on salads, or to cook up to 350°F or 180°C)

Anyone not quite ready to give up packaged foods and fast-food restaurants can for now increase their fish oil intake, both through diet and with supplements—ensuring the origin and quality!

Again, it's the relationship and not the absolute amount of fatty acids that's important to our health. The more natural, unprocessed products we eat, the closer we get to the original healthy ratio.

SUPER FUEL: SHORT AND MEDIUM CHAIN FATTY ACIDS

Short and medium chain fatty acids have so many positive effects because they are differently metabolized than the long chain acids. Medium chain fatty acids do not need bile to be present in the stomach in order to be absorbed. After digestion in the stomach they go directly to the intestines, and from there straight into the blood.

Short and medium chain fatty acids:

- Stimulate the metabolism
- Are effective against many viruses, certain bacteria, and fungi
- Increase energy levels and performance
- Are easy to digest
- Are satiating and keep blood sugar stable
- Strengthen the immune system

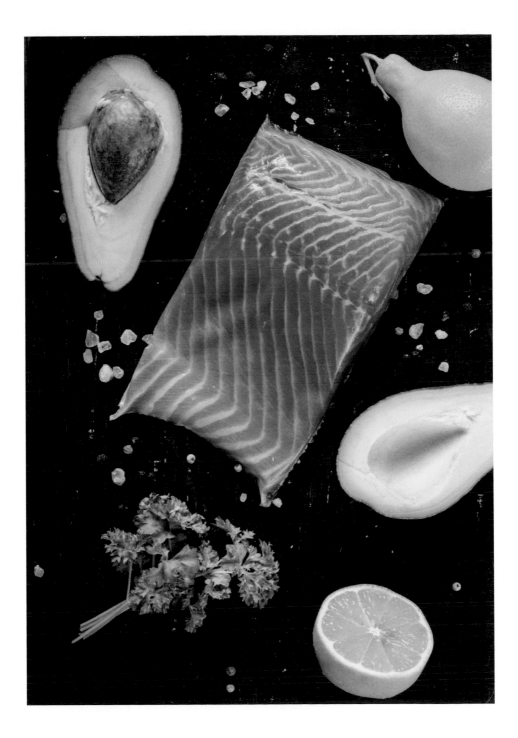

BODY FAT
WHAT IS THE BODY COMPOSITION OF A HEALTHY HUMAN?

A healthy middle-aged man is on average approximately 50 to 60 percent water, 15 percent body fat, 10 percent bones, and 20 to 30 percent muscle. In women, the natural body fat percentage is slightly higher, at about 20 percent, and the bone and muscle mass are correspondingly a little lower.

There is nothing wrong if the body fat percentage is somewhat higher than mentioned above, when the fat mass is distributed relatively evenly over the body. It's fat deposits in the abdominal area, in and around the organs, that are unhealthy.

.

DR. TORSTEN ALBERS
HOW MUCH BODY FAT IS HEALTHY?

The WHO defines a body mass index (BMI) from 25 to 30 as overweight and over 30 as obese. The BMI is easy to calculate; the only numbers needed for calculation are height and weight, both easily determined. BMI does *not* distinguish between increased body fat and increased muscle mass—those with a lot of weight from muscle will get a high BMI value.

Body fat percentage, on the other hand, refers to the amount of body fat as a percentage of total body weight. This measurement is far more difficult to obtain, and in reality a person's body fat is never 100 percent accurately measurable. Underwater weighing and DEXA are the most reliable methods for determining body fat today.

The DEXA measurement uses X-rays (with a radiation dose lower than you'd receive during air travel!). Conclusions about body fat, muscle, and bone mass are then drawn based on absorption of X-rays. Such DEXA devices are very expensive and available only in a few specialized centers. It would be challenging to screen large populations in order to determine normal values of body fat percentage, compared to using the BMI. Therefore, there is no good scientifically based and validated data for the reference ranges for body fat in men or women, let alone children and teens, approved by professional medical associations.

Other techniques for the measurement of body fat, such as the bio-impedance measurement (e.g., "fat measuring scales") or the skin-fold measurement using calipers, are far less accurate, and in the second case depend a lot on the person doing the measuring. Furthermore, the data of skin-fold measurements used to calculate the body-fat percentage usually gives numbers 3 to 4 percentage points lower than the results of accurate DEXA measurement (e.g., 16 percent instead of 19 to 20 percent with DEXA).

For these reasons, the following table is only a guideline for the assessment of the body fat percentage value of a person. It is based essentially on the experience of the authors, as well as the small amount of data available from studies.

Assessment of body fat values of a person, determined with DEXA

	Very Low Professional athlete	**Low** Well-trained person	**Average**	**High** Health at risk	**Considerably increased** Alarmingly high health risk
Men	< 10 %	10–15 %	15–22 %	22–30 %	> 30 %
Women	< 14 %	13–20 %	20–30 %	30–38 %	> 38 %

In women, very low values of less than 12 percent will often lead to loss of menstruation and, in the long run, loss of bone mass (osteoporosis)—so it's important to stay in the healthy range or only slightly below most of the time.

HOW HIGH SHOULD THE PROPORTION OF FAT IN THE DIET BE?

How much fat or oil should you be eating to maintain a healthy body fat percentage?

1. More important than the absolute amount of fat we eat is choosing the right healthy fats and oils.
2. We must eat more healthy fats and oils than the low-fat advocates have told us we should over the past few decades.
3. In addition to the correct choice of fats and oils, starchy carbohydrates (cereals, bread, pasta, potatoes, etc.) and sugar should be avoided. All carbohydrates and sugar that we do not burn are stored in fat deposits.
4. Healthy fats and oils do not make you fat. Superfluous carbohydrates are, however, stored in fat deposits.

PURE FOOD—FAT-FRIENDLY NUTRITION

PRINCIPLES

PRINCIPLE 1
Eat natural foods. A good way to choose your menu is to only eat foods you could consume raw—vegetables, fruits, meat, fish, eggs, nuts, seeds, water, and raw milk. We avoid anything that we couldn't eat raw (cereals, potatoes, legumes, etc.).

I'm not saying you have to eat raw, just that foods we are able to eat raw are well tolerated. Cooking food makes it easier to digest, tastier, and the nutrients more easily absorbed and can help you vary your diet.

PRINCIPLE 2
Buy unprocessed food—no artificial additives such as flavorings, thickeners, and colorings. All artificial additives interfere with our natural satiety signals and food instinct. A good example is artificial sugars. Although they do not contain calories, they trigger hunger and appetite. That is why they're used in animal feed—to make the animals eat more than they would naturally.

PRINCIPLE 3
Eat, whenever possible, local food. The transport routes are shorter and the environment becomes less polluted. We buy directly from the farmers or producers, and find out firsthand how the animals are treated and whether the fruit and veggies are really organic.

PRINCIPLE 4
Eat, whenever possible, seasonal local food. The nutrient density of ripe, freshly harvested fruit and vegetables is higher than from immature-harvested or hydroponically grown vegetables and fruits. Eating seasonal veggies and fruit automatically diversifies our menu.

PRINCIPLE 5
Eat, whenever possible, organically grown vegetables, fruits, and animal products. The science is still inconclusive about whether organic produce has more nutrients than conventionally farmed produce, but obviously organic farming uses fewer pesticides. This damages nature less, and the food you eat isn't covered with poisons.

In animal products, the organic label guarantees that the animals have been humanely reared and fed well. This is very important to us—on the one hand for the benefit of animals, and on the other hand, because the meat, fish, poultry, and eggs are much more nutritious. We can only stay healthy if we're eating healthy food.

Food contaminated with manufactured fertilizers and antibiotics does humans no good. And meat from animals fattened with grains contains an unnatural composition of fatty acids—not good for humans either!

PRINCIPLE 6

Pure Food balances nutrients. The macronutrients are evenly divided into about 30 percent proteins, 30 percent carbohydrates, and 40 percent fat.

We attach great importance to consuming enough healthy fats. As you've learned, fat does not make you fat. Excess carbohydrates are being stored in your fat deposits.

In the Pure Food diet, fat comes from the following foods: meat, fish, poultry, eggs, avocado, virgin coconut oil, butter, ghee, nuts, and a little extra-virgin olive oil. Apart from the nuts and the olive oil, these fats contain either no or very few omega-6 fatty acids. Avoid vegetable fats, as they include sunflower or peanut oil. These fats are highly processed and quickly become rancid. Most of these industrially processed oils contain high amounts of omega-6 fatty acids, which lead to a poor ratio of omega-6s to omega-3s.

PRINCIPLE 7

Eat gluten-free. Gluten, a protein in some grains, is difficult to digest. Often it is not completely broken down into individual amino acids, and incompletely digested gluten fragments, called peptides, remain. Depending on the condition of the intestinal mucosa, they can pass through the mucosa (as in leaky gut syndrome) and be released into the bloodstream. Gluten peptides can also trigger allergic reactions, consisting of swelling and inflammation. Unlike an insect bite on your arm, where the swelling is easily recognizable and palpable, you might not necessarily feel the swelling in the intestines triggered by an allergic reaction to food.

Even more difficult to recognize is allergic inflammation in the brain. The brain tissue cannot, unlike your skin, make itself itchy, painful, or swollen. Therefore, extended allergic inflammation in the brain—for example, due to gluten peptides—is very subtle, with symptoms like a "foggy head" feeling.

Grains contain no essential nutrients and can be removed from the diet without any problems.

PRINCIPLE 8

Reduce sugar intake to a minimum. Not just table sugar, but all kinds of sugar, including honey, fructose, maple syrup, and all artificial sugars. The less sugar we consume, the more sensitive our taste buds are. Our cravings for sweets diminish and natural sweetness tastes better again.

I am absolutely not a fan of artificial sugar substitutes. It's ridiculous for food manufacturers to sell them as a healthy alternative to sugar. If we eat artificial sugars, our brains continue to be addicted to sugar, and we won't be satisfied with natural foods. Sugar is an addictive substance, like alcohol, heroin, nicotine, and other drugs.

If you feel truly desperate for sweets, then eat small amounts of dark chocolate (good quality, without artificial additives and with a minimum of 72 percent cocoa), fruits, or homemade desserts sweetened with minimal sugar, and enjoy them consciously, without overindulging.

PRINCIPLE 9

Eat and drink raw dairy products whenever possible. Dairy products are, unfortunately, destroyed by pasteurization and homogenization. The human body cannot properly identify and digest what is coming into the stomach—some kind of new combination of water and milk fat without any enzymes or bacteria. In raw milk, water and milk fat are separated—you can see this process when cream rises to the top in a bottle of raw milk you put in the refrigerator.

Raw milk in its original state, i.e., as it flows directly from the udder of a cow, can be better digested by many people. There are several reasons for this. The enzymes in raw milk are not destroyed by heating (pasteurization) and can actively support the human digestive process. In homogenization, the water and fat in the milk are combined. Thus, the cream cannot settle on the top of milk. The milk is always the same. The disadvantage of the "beautiful," uniform, homogenized milk is that our systems just can't digest it; it can cause bloating, diarrhea, abdominal cramps, constipation, chronic inflammation in the intestines, and other ailments.

It should be noted that not everyone can digest raw milk and raw-milk products (raw butter, raw-milk cheese, etc.). A lack of lactase (a digestive enzyme in the stomach) or an intolerance to casein (milk protein) are unfortunately relatively common.

Lactose intolerance shows up with an elimination diet: Get rid of all dairy products for a week and see how you feel, then reintroduce them and see if you feel worse. Faster, but also less reliable, is a test that your doctor can perform.

PRINCIPLE 10

Avoid legumes because they are hard to digest. The composition of macronutrients (fat, protein, and carbohydrates) in legumes is not optimal. Legumes contain little protein and many carbohydrates and anti-nutrients. These are lectins and saponins, which make the intestinal walls permeable (i.e., leaky gut syndrome) and trigger chronic inflammation in the body.

FINALLY

These recommendations are not stubborn and fanatical. The longer you eat according to these principles, the more effortlessly you'll be able to navigate eating in everyday life, at the weekend, at parties, on vacation.

It's very important to be strict with food that can make you sick even with the smallest quantities, such as in celiac disease, where even tiny traces of gluten can cause severe symptoms.

With children, be gentle and try not to cause permanent damage with a shift in diet! At home, keep only Pure Foods. Offer a big selection of healthy foods and let children decide for themselves what they want to eat. This makes less hassle for you, and if the kids aren't fussing, everyone will digest their food better.

Children should be part of the shopping and cooking whenever possible, which will increase the likelihood that they'll eat what they see on the table.

The adults have to make good decisions when shopping. Study so-called children's food labels closely! There's often a lot of unhealthy ingredients, like sugar, fructose, and trans fats. Parents are responsible for ensuring that such foods are unavailable at home. If the fridge and pantry at home are full of junk food, of course kids will crave it from an early age.

Going away and eating out with children is slightly more difficult. The wide range of tempting products (especially the countless heavily sugared products) can be overwhelming. Children often do not understand why they should resist temptation. They also often feel no direct negative effect from the consumption of harmful foods. We parents see it—the children are hyperactive, have allergies, eczema, lack of concentration, a runny nose and much more.

Young people need natural products full of flavor and nutrients to be healthy, happy, and intelligent.

MEAL PLANS: PRACTICAL IMPLEMENTATION OF THE PURE FOOD DIET

IMPLEMENTATION

1   These meal plans are intended as inspiration.
2.   Each main meal can be substituted. It does not matter if you're eating a dish for breakfast, lunch, or dinner.
3.   The snacks are optional. Only snack if you're actually hungry between meals.
4   If you eat a dessert, make sure you eat it right after the main meal. This is very important with fruits, which should always be eaten with protein and fat so that the fructose doesn't stimulate insulin production followed by ravenous hunger.
5   Each main meal, including dessert, is balanced. That is, about 30 percent protein, 30 percent carbohydrates, and 40 percent fat. Likewise, the whole day is balanced.

SERVING SIZE

*   The Pure Food approach does not count calories or maintain rigid portion sizes.
*   Maintaining the balance of macronutrients is important:
    *   30 percent of the calories are from protein-containing foods.
    *   30 percent of the calories are carbohydrates of gluten-free foods.
    *   40 percent of the calories are from the recommended fats and oils.

To facilitate your journey into the Pure Food diet, I have provided many meal plans. This includes dishes with the recipes listed later and simple meals that you can cook yourself or order in a restaurant.

The following meal plans are calculated for a person who is about 145 lbs and 5'5". For a person of this build, you could divide the recipes into four—of course, if the people eating are bigger, then the recipes would divide better into three.

For snacks, eat only enough to tide you over until the next main meal.

Anyone much smaller or larger, heavier or lighter, can correspondingly eat smaller or larger portions, always maintaining the macronutrient breakdown of 30 percent protein, 30 percent carbs, and 40 percent fat.

CHILDREN

Children can eat this diet as well as adults. Give a child smaller portions and allow her to eat what she likes. As long as she is eating natural food, her body intelligence will signal to her how much and what to eat. There will be days when a child eats many more carbohydrates and other days only meat. Even serving size will vary from day to day and from meal to meal. Never force a child to clean her plate, but also don't spoil her appetite with sweets between meals.

BEVERAGES
- Water is the most important thirst quencher.
- Completely avoid all soft drinks, energy drinks, and fruit juices.
- Two or three cups of high-quality coffee or black or green tea before lunch are okay—no caffeinated beverages after lunch.
- Ginger tea and herbal tea can be drunk as desired.
- One to two glasses of good wine can be drunk now and then, if you are satisfied with your weight and are not trying to lose pounds.

Note: In mealtime plans the calories are listed so that we can calculate the distribution of macronutrients. Calorie numbers always depend on product and quality; therefore, these figures are only an approximation and not precise data.

PURE FOOD IN THE RESTAURANT

If a restaurant has a menu online, read it and decide which items you can eat and might want before you visit—being prepared will help you stay strong in the face of unhealthy temptations.

1. Don't feel embarrassed about asking how the food is cooked at the restaurant:
   - Is the sauce gluten-free?
   - Is the food fried in sunflower seed oil?
   - Is the fish breaded?

2. Politely ask for accommodations:
   - Can I have the fish grilled without breading and some more salad or veggies?
   - Can I please have the fish grilled instead of baked?
   - Please bring me the salad without dressing. I'd like to have oil and vinegar to make my own dressing at the table.
   - Please don't bring a bread basket (or please take the bread basket away).
   - I'm sorry, I don't see anything I can eat on the menu; is it possible for you to make me a vegetable omelette fried in olive oil?

WHAT CAN YOU EXPECT?
MORE ENERGY AND VITALITY

Your blood sugar will be stable and constant throughout the day.

You'll have fewer sugar cravings, and they'll disappear completely in time.

With a balanced diet, all of your nutritional needs are covered. Your hormonal system will regulate itself naturally and function optimally again. This will make you happier and more balanced.

In the evening, you'll fall into a healthy, deep sleep and wake up in the morning fresh and ready to go, ensuring you'll be mentally and physically capable.

Anyone carrying around a little too much body fat will reduce it without starving.

Because you'll have more energy you'll also be able to incorporate strength training and exercise into everyday life.

Muscles give you strength and a nice shape.

PURE FOOD –
HEALTHY, SLENDER, AND SATISFIED.

MEAL PLANS

Recipes that are listed later in the book are marked with green.

PURE FOOD MEAL PLANS (EASY TO COOK)			
Day	**Monday**	**Tuesday**	**Wednesday**
Breakfast	Coconut-Blueberry Smoothie	2 eggs hard-boiled 0.7 oz (20 g) mayonnaise 7 oz (200 g) fruit (for example melon)	1 serving leftover dinner from Tuesday
Snack	1.4 oz (40 g) Paleo beef jerky and cherry tomatoes	10 macadamia nuts (0.7 oz, or 20 g)	1 hard-boiled egg with salt
Lunch	5.2 oz (150 g) fish fillet grilled (e.g., cod) 0.7 oz (20 g) herb butter 3.5 oz (100 g) leafy greens with 1 tbsp olive oil	5.2 oz (150 g) burger without bun (fried egg and/or 2 strips of bacon, optional) with mixed salad leaves	Sardine Salad
Snack/Dessert	1 oz (30 g) Chocolate-Nut Butter 3.5 oz (100 g) apple slices	7 oz (200 g) fresh berries	About 0.7 oz (20 g) chocolate (72 percent cocoa)
Dinner	Grilled chicken, 5.2 oz (150 g) steamed spinach	Pork Chops with Asian Salad	Unbreaded Cordon Bleu with spinach
Dessert	1 serving Chocolate Mousse	2 Coconut Macaroons	1 small banana (4.2 oz or 120 g)
Total calories 143 lbs / 5'5" (65 kg / 170 cm) 165 / 5'9" (75 kg / 180 cm)	1620 1770	1830 1980	1350 1500
Nutrient chart			

● CARBOHYDRATES ● PROTEIN ● FAT

PURE FOOD MEAL PLANS (EASY TO COOK)

Thursday	Friday	Saturday	Sunday
Avocado Smoothie	1 serving leftover dinner from Thursday	Smoothie with Egg	Cheese Omelette with spinach Fried Bacon with Popovers
6 olives 1 oz (30 g) ham	10 walnuts (0.7 oz or 20 g)	1.7 oz (50 g) cooked chicken breast and cucumber	
Caesar Salad with chicken breast (without sweet potatoes or no dessert)	salad of 7 oz (200 g) broccoli 2 eggs 1 oz (30 g) mayonnaise	Fish tartare with salad leaves	
1 small banana	1.4 oz (40 g) Paleo beef jerky and pickles	10 macadamia nuts (0.7 oz or 20 g)	Baked Fish in foil 3.5 oz (100 g) pumpkin 3.5 oz (100 g) zucchini 3.5 oz (100 g) carrots
Merguez with vegetables	Muesli from 1.4 oz (40 g) Chocolate-Nut Butter 7 oz (200 g) skim raw-milk cheese 1 small banana	Paleo Curry with beef	
2 Almond-Chocolate Biscotti		5.2 oz (150 g) papaya	1 serving Coconut Pudding
1580	1800	1920	1360
1730	1950	2070	1510

MEAL PLANS

Recipes listed later in the book are marked with green.

PURE FOOD MEAL PLANS (SLIGHTLY MORE COMPLICATED RECIPES)			
Day	**Monday**	**Tuesday**	**Wednesday**
Breakfast	Coconut-Banana Smoothie	1 serving Muesli plus 7 oz (200 g) raw-milk quark	Cheese Omelette with Parmesan and tomatoes 7 oz (200 g) grapes
Snack	1.4 oz (40 g) Paleo beef jerky and cherry tomatoes	1 hard-boiled egg with salt	6 olives 1 oz (30 g) ham
Lunch	Caesar salad with grilled chicken breast (without sweet potatoes, or no dessert)	5.2 oz (150 g) fish fillet (e.g., sea bass, trout) 0.7 oz (20 g) herb butter steamed vegetables	5.2 oz (150 g) burger without a bun (2 strips of fried bacon optional) with 2.6 oz (75 g) fries
Snack/Dessert	1 small banana	10 macadamia nuts (0.7 oz or 20 g)	0.7 oz (20 g) chocolate (72 percent cocoa)
Dinner	Sweet Potato Chips with Beef Tartare	Oriental Lamb Stew with zucchini	Rice Noodles with Carbonara Sauce
Dessert	1 Almond-Chocolate Biscotti	1 serving of Chocolate Mousse	7 oz (200 g) strawberries
Total calories **143 lbs / 5'5"** **(65 kg / 170 cm)** **165 / 5'9"** **(75 kg / 180 cm)**	1570 1720	1700 1850	2030 2180
Nutrient chart			

● CARBOHYDRATES ● PROTEIN ● FAT

PURE FOOD MEAL PLANS (SLIGHTLY MORE COMPLICATED RECIPES)

Thursday	Friday	Saturday	Sunday
Avocado Smoothie	1 serving leftover dinner from Thursday	Fried Bacon with Popovers	
1.7 oz (50 g) cooked chicken breast and cucumber	10 Macadamia nuts (0.7 oz or 20 g)	10 walnuts (0.7 oz or 20 g)	Coconut Kaiserschmarrn with 1 egg
Schnitzel Rolls with Tapenade Filling and steamed vegetables 1 tbsp butter or olive oil	Unbreaded Cordon Bleu with 7 oz (200 g) spinach steamed	Fish tartare with salad leaves	1/2 avocado 3 strips fried bacon
1 peach	0.7 oz (20 g) chocolate (72 percent cocoa)	5.2 oz (150 g) blueberries	
Duck Breast with broccoli 7 oz (200 g)	Apple with Nut Filling	Thai Veal Shank with mashed potatoes	Liver Saltimbocca with Butternut Squash
1 piece Olive Oil Cake (1/10 of the whole cake)	1 oz (30 g) raw-milk cheese (e.g., Parmesan)	1 serving Cinnamon-Coconut Ice Cream	Chocolate Pavlova with Cocoa Quark Cream (1/2 meal)
1680	1440	1910	1400
1830	1590	2060	1550

45

KETOGENIC DIET—HIGH-FAT NUTRITION

PRINCIPLES

Apply the same principles as the Pure Food diet (pages 34-37), with some differences in the distribution of macronutrients.

In a ketogenic diet, carbohydrates and protein content are greatly reduced. The body is forced to generate its energy from fat and body fat deposits.

DR. TORSTEN ALBERS
WHEN IS A KETOGENIC DIET USEFUL?

Many people think the ketogenic or Atkins diet is just for losing weight. In clinical nutrition, however, this diet has long been used as a therapeutic measure in children with epilepsy. The elevated levels of ketone bodies in the blood prevent the occurrence of seizures very reliably if the fat intake is kept permanently at about 90 percent of total calories, which represents an extremely high fat component, only achievable with an abundant supply of foods like butter, cream, and macadamia nuts. Long-term studies in children and adolescents who suffer from epilepsy show that these individuals don't suffer any harm in later adulthood caused by this diet that so widely differs from the official recommendations.

Another topic of debate is how a ketogenic diet would be useful in cancer patients. Since up to 40 percent of patients do not die from the tumor itself, but from malnutrition and physical wasting, we have to consider how we might mitigate this process. Since cancer patients can metabolize carbohydrates only very poorly in the muscle cells but can metabolize fats very well, there are now studies underway to see if a protein- and fat-rich diet could possibly be helpful here. Initial results show that a ketogenic diet improves the nutritional status of patients with very aggressive tumor types, leads to weight increase or stops weight loss, lessens muscle weakness, and improves long-term prognosis and mortality rates.

In otherwise healthy individuals who have elevated sugar and insulin levels, do little to no physical activity, and want to lose weight very quickly, this form of diet can make particular sense. In this case, the increased insulin levels are significantly reduced by the very low number of carbohydrates, and the fat loss is usually quicker than with a higher carbohydrate intake. Due to the high fat intake, the body will be forced to also increasingly rev up the metabolic processes of fat burning. Finally, a strong appetite suppression comes with a strictly ketogenic diet. This will lead to a significantly lowered caloric intake. Thus, the body covers the resulting energy deficit with the body's store of fat.

The switch to a low-carbohydrate diet can mean a big change for the body in the first one to three weeks. This can go along with mild to severe fatigue, sugar cravings, headaches, mild flu symptoms, and sometimes mood swings (in our experience more in women than in men).

IMPLEMENTATION

1. The meals plans are intended as inspiration.
2. Each main meal can be substituted. It doesn't matter if you're eating these meals for breakfast, lunch, or dinner.
3. The snacks are optional. Only eat them if you're actually hungry between meals.
4. Fruits contain a lot of fructose and are therefore not eaten on a ketogenic diet.
5. The macronutrients are balanced as 75 to 85 percent fat, 10 to 15 percent protein, and 5 to 10 percent carbohydrates.
6. Once a week, start eating carbs in the afternoon and for dinner. Fats are reduced for these meals. This is called carb loading, and it's important in rebalancing the satiety hormone leptin.

CARB LOADING

The morning after carb loading, you might find you weigh a few pounds more. That's because the increased intake of carbohydrates leads to water retention. This is natural and will disappear after one to three days. The water retention is usually more pronounced in women than in men.

Don't let it deter you from carb loading!

In order to avoid heaviness, bloating, and fatigue, you should eat gluten-free carbs, like bananas, sweet potatoes, potatoes, or white rice.

Carb loading within the ketogenic diet (one high-carb meal every seven to ten days) is only necessary for healthy and active people to lose fat until their desired weight is reached. Then they can switch to a balanced Pure Food diet.

Those who live with conditions such as epilepsy or illnesses such as cancer should not carb load. It is advisable to seek advice from a doctor before you start with a ketogenic diet.

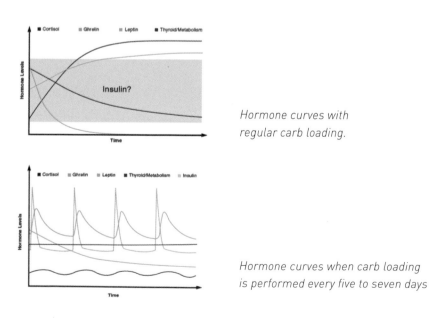

Hormone curves with
regular carb loading.

Hormone curves when carb loading
is performed every five to seven days

DR. TORSTEN ALBERS
AVOIDING LOSS OF MUSCLE MASS

Keeping muscle while losing a lot of body fat is more difficult while on a ketogenic diet, because the stress hormone cortisol promotes loss of muscle mass by its catabolic effects in the body. The lack of a regular insulin surge "charging" the muscles with carbohydrates after training supports the muscle breakdown processes in the long run. The leptin signal from the fat cells decreases even further without "loading days" and will promote cravings and a decrease in basal metabolic rate.

SERVING SIZE

- Don't count calories or use strict portion control.
- To maintain a ketogenic state you **must** adhere to the macronutrient balance:
    - 10 to 15 percent of calories are from protein-containing foods.
    - 5 to 10 percent of calories are carbohydrates from gluten-free foods.
    - 75 to 85 percent are from the recommended fats and oils.

Note: Not only are carbohydrates greatly reduced in the ketogenic diet, but so are proteins. Proteins are converted into glucose, like carbs. Fats, however, are converted into ketones.

BURNING PROTEIN

If you want to lose weight, of course you want to reduce body fat and not muscle. To make sure that's what you're doing, your body needs to be able to burn fat from food or fat from your body for energy—another reason not to replace the carbohydrates with proteins, since protein can also be converted to glucose and used as an energy carrier.

It makes perfect sense—nature stores excess energy in our body as fat rather than protein. Therefore, it is much more sensible to use the fuel designed for us by nature. And that's fat.

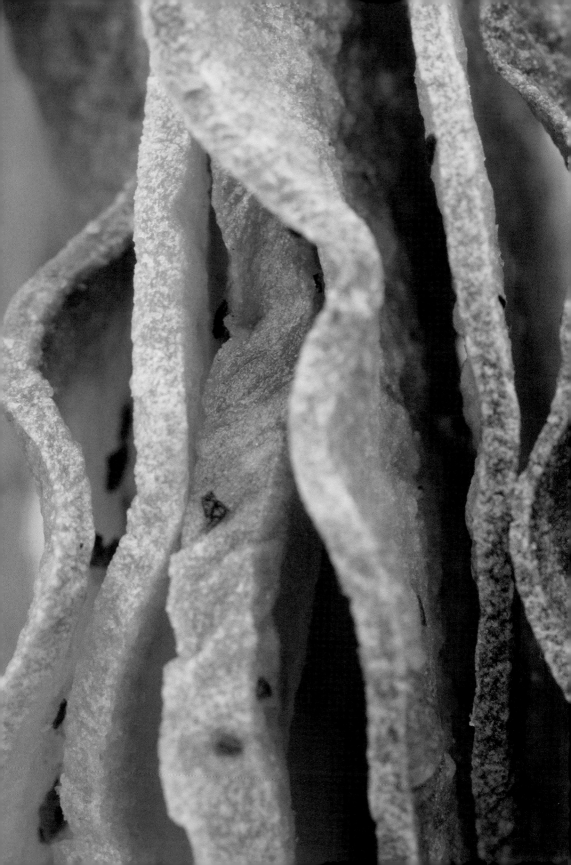

The following meal plans are calculated for a person who is about 145 lbs or 5'5". For a person of this build, you could divide the recipes into four—of course, if a person is bigger, then the recipes would divide better into three.

Only eat snacks to tide you over till your next meal.

If you're shorter or taller, heavier or lighter, you can eat correspondingly smaller or larger portions. Always observe the distribution of the macronutrients of 10 to 15 percent protein, 5 to 10 percent carbohydrates, and 75 to 85 percent fat.

KETOGENIC MEAL PLANS

Recipes that are listed later in the book are marked with green.

KETOGENIC NUTRITIONAL MEAL PLANS			
Day	**Monday**	**Tuesday**	**Wednesday**
Breakfast	2 eggs, hard-boiled 1/2 avocado 0.7 oz (20 g) mayonnaise	Butter Coffee (coffee with 0.7 oz or 20 g of butter)	1 serving leftover dinner from Tuesday
Snack	1.4 oz (40 g) Italian salami with 3.5 oz (100 g) cherry tomatoes	5 olives with 1 oz (30 g) ham	1 hard-boiled egg with 0.7 oz (20 g) mayonnaise
Lunch	5.2 oz (150 g) schnitzel (pork) grilled with 0.7 oz (20 g) herb butter 3.5 oz (100 g) salad leaves 2 tbsp olive oil	5.2 oz (150 g) of tuna in olive oil, 3.5 oz (100 g) salad leaves	5.2 oz (150 g) burger without bun, 3.5 oz (100 g) lettuce 1 tbsp olive oil (1 fried egg and 3 fried bacon strips optional)
Snack/Dessert	10 macadamia nuts (0.7 oz or 20 g)	0.4 oz (10 g) chocolate (72 percent cocoa)	0.4 oz (10 g) chocolate (72 percent cocoa)
Dinner	Grilled chicken with skin 5.2 oz (150 g) steamed spinach 1 tbsp butter	Pork Chops with Asian Salad	Sardines in olive oil with green salad
Dessert	0.4 oz (10 g) chocolate (72 percent cocoa)	1 oz (30 g) full-fat cheese from raw milk, 0.5 oz (5 g) butter	1 oz (30 g) nut butter 2.8 oz (80 g) full-fat raw cream cheese
Total calories 143 lbs / 5'5" (65 kg / 170 cm) 165 / 5'9" (75 kg / 180 cm)	1980 2130	1310 1460	2000 2150
Nutrient chart			

● CARBOHYDRATES ● PROTEIN ● FAT

KETOGENIC NUTRITIONAL MEAL PLANS

Thursday	Friday	Saturday	Sunday
2 eggs in 1 avocado	1 serving of leftover dinner from Thursday	Coconut Coffee (coffee and 0.7 oz or 20 g of coconut oil)	Cheese Omelette with spinach 5 strips fried bacon, and 7 oz (200 g) tomatoes
5 olives 1 oz (30 g) ham	1 egg hard-boiled 0.7 oz (20 g) mayonnaise	1 oz (30 g) salami 3.5 oz (100 g) cucumber	
Caesar Salad with shrimp (without sweet potatoes)	Chicken thighs with skin and 3.5 oz (100 g) salad leaves 2 tbsp olive oil	7 oz (200 g) broccoli 2 eggs hard-boiled 1 oz (30 g) mayonnaise	
10 walnuts (0.7 oz or 20 g)	10 macadamia nuts (0.7 oz or 20 g)	10 walnuts (0.7 oz or 20 g)	1–2 banana and chocolate (72 percent cocoa)
Merguez with 5.2 oz (150 g) cauliflower 1 tbsp butter	Unbreaded Cordon Bleu 5 .2 oz (150 g) broccoli 1 tbsp butter	4.4 oz (125 g) salmon fillet 3.5 oz (100 g) salad leaves 2 tbsp olive oil	7 oz (200 g) curry dish plus 7 oz (200g) cooked rice or 7 oz (200 g) of potatoes
1 oz (30 g) raw-milk cheese full-fat (e.g., Gruyère) with 0.5 oz (15 g) butter	0.4 oz (10 g) chocolate (72 percent cocoa)	1 serving Chocolate Mousse	Coconut pudding
1520	1810	1560	at least 1750
1670	1960	1710	at least 1900

FAT SOURCES

AVOCADO

The avocado is native to Central and South America. It has been cultivated since about 8000 BC. Today the fatty fruit is grown in almost all tropical and sub-tropical countries.

The avocado belongs to the laurel family and is the fattiest fruit of all, with approximately 85 percent fat content.

There are around four hundred varieties grown worldwide. In many places, the creamy Hass avocado is the most popular. Avocados are always immature-picked from the tree and ripen after. The Hass avocado ripens from green to black. It is deliciously ripe when the shell gives way to light finger pressure.

The fat of the avocado has anti-inflammatory properties that help the body heal inflammation. This effect is well documented, for example in arthritis sufferers.

RECIPES

In these featured recipes I use Hass avocados. Each avocado has an average of 5.6 oz (160 g) of edible pulp.

AN AVOCADO IS RIPE WHEN THE SHELL GIVES WAY TO LIGHT FINGER PRESSURE.

In order for these recipes to work, you have to use ripe avocados. Because there are often only unripe avocados in grocery stores, it's worthwhile to buy them regularly, so you always have avocados in various stages of maturity at home.

If an avocado is ripe but I'm not ready to eat it, I put it in the refrigerator, where its ripening will slow considerably.

AVOCADO FATTY ACID PROFILE

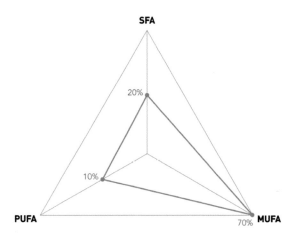

SFA

SFA

20%

10%

PUFA

70% MUFA

SFA = saturated fatty acids

PUFA = polyunsaturated fatty acids

MUFA = monounsaturated fatty acids

BASIL GUACAMOLE

1 ripe avocado
bunch of basil
   (approximately 1 cup
   of leaves packed)
1 tsp (5 ml) sambal
   oelek
salt
pepper

GUACAMOLE VARIATIONS

PREPARATION

Cut the avocado in the middle lengthwise,
remove the stone, loosen the flesh from the shell, and place in a bowl.
Pluck the basil leaves, wash, dry, finely chop, and add to the bowl.
Add sambal oelek and finely mash with a fork until no solid pieces remain.
Season with salt and pepper.

SERVING SUGGESTIONS

Works very well with fried or grilled meat or as a dip
with vegetable sticks or chips.

WASABI GUACAMOLE

Switch out cilantro for the basil and replace sambal oelek with
1 tsp (5 ml) wasabi paste.

MANGO GUACAMOLE

Leave out the basil and replace the sambal oelek with
1 small fresh red chili, finely chopped.
Crush together with the avocado.
Once this is done, stir in 3.5 oz (100 g) of mango,
peeled and cut into small cubes.

Excellent with grilled shrimp or fish fillet.

AVOCADO SALAD DRESSING

PREPARATION

Cut the avocado in half lengthwise, remove the stone, and loosen the flesh from the shell. Cut into pieces and place in a mixing bowl.

Add lemon juice and olive oil to the bowl and mix well into a sauce with an electric mixer or a food processor.

Wash, dry, and finely chop the herbs, then mix with the sauce. Add water or vegetable broth until the dressing is liquid enough for you. Season with salt and pepper.

.

SERVING SUGGESTIONS

Ideal for vegetables and green salads.

Tuna Salad: Mix drained tinned tuna and Avocado Salad Dressing well. Serve with green salad.

.

4-6 SALAD SERVINGS

....

1 ripe avocado
1 tbsp (15 ml) lemon juice
3-6 tbsp (50-100 ml) extra-virgin olive oil
salt
pepper
1 bunch fresh herbs
(e.g., cilantro, basil, chives)
vegetable stock or water
to dilute the sauce a bit (optional)

AVOCADO SMOOTHIE

---------------------------- **PREPARATION** ----------------------------

Cut all the fruit into pieces and place in a blender.
Add milk, if desired, and a portion of the water, as well as the protein powder or gelatin, and blend until it's completely homogenous.

If you're using vanilla extract, add now with a little water or ice.

---------------------------- **STORAGE** ----------------------------

Drink straight away, as avocados brown quickly.

1 mini-banana (about 1.5 oz or 50 g), peeled
3.5 oz (100 g) mango, peeled
avocado (approximately 2.8 oz or 80 g)
approximately 0.8 cups (200 ml) water
or appropriate amount of ice
0.4–0.8 cups (100–200 ml) raw milk
(optional instead of water)
1 oz (30 g) protein powder or instant gelatin
1 tsp (5 ml) vanilla extract or powder (optional)

EGG IN AVOCADO

PREPARATION

Preheat the oven to 350°F (180°C).

Cut the avocado in half lengthwise, remove the stone, and carefully spoon out a little bit of the avocado to make the center hole bigger for the egg.

Pour an egg into each hole. Sprinkle the Parmesan over the eggs and cook 15 minutes in the oven.

Ideally, the egg white and the yolk should still be slightly liquid. The cooking time will vary from oven to oven.

Before serving, sprinkle with paprika and salt.

SERVING SUGGESTIONS

For a balanced meal, serve with a green salad and some fried chicken breast.

ALTERNATIVE

Poach a quail egg and then place in the hole of an avocado sliced in half lengthwise. Sprinkle with Parmesan, paprika, and salt.

1–2 SERVINGS

1 ripe avocado
2 small organic eggs
0.7 oz (20 g) Parmesan, freshly grated
salt
paprika

6-7 DESSERT SERVINGS

2 ripe avocados
2 ripe bananas
1 oz (30 g) cocoa powder (not chocolate powder!)
1 oz (30 g) honey (optional)
1 tsp (5 ml) cinnamon, ground (optional)
1 tsp (5 ml) vanilla, crushed (optional)

CHOCOLATE CREAM

PREPARATION

Puree all the ingredients in a bowl or jug with a hand blender
until no lumps are present.

SERVING SUGGESTIONS

Pour the cream into small dessert bowls and garnish with banana slices.

SHELF LIFE

Eat immediately!

COCONUT

Coconuts provide a clear, pure oil with a mild, fine, nutty, and aromatic flavor. Coconut oil melts at about 77°F (25°C). It is solid at refrigerator temperature and creamy at room temperature.

In countries where it's indigenous, the oil is used for cooking, frying, deep frying, and for skin and hair care.

The term "virgin" applied to coconut oil indicates that it is produced only by cold-pressing. The best quality oil comes from small family-owned organic farms, in which the organic coconuts are harvested by hand. After gentle drying, the meat of the nuts is crushed. The resulting shredded coconut is then subjected to a gentle cold-pressing. Thus extracted, high-quality organic coconut oil only needs to be filtered and bottled.

After extraction of the high-quality oil, squeezed coconut meat remains. It is rich in nutrients and fiber and can supplement a sensible diet in the form of coconut flour. It is low in carbohydrates and gluten-free.

PURE VIRGIN COCONUT OIL:

- Is easy to digest
- Contains no harmful trans fats
- Contains no cholesterol
- Enhances the good cholesterol already in the body
- Contains many medium chain fatty acids, especially lauric acid
- Is a good source of selenium
- Protects against bacteria, viruses, and fungi
- Has a long shelf life
- Is versatile (e.g., body cream, oil pulling)
- Is a good substitute for butter for those with a milk allergy

INDUSTRIAL PRODUCTION PROCESS

The method and the quality of industrially produced coconut oil are quite different from the product produced with cold-pressing. The coconut meat is dried in the sun outdoors. In many places it is simply dumped on the roadside, polluted by the exhaust of passing cars and often moldy because of the tropical humidity. The smoke-drying process is faster. It can, however, lead to undesirably high levels of pollutants. Heat is then used to squeeze the oil out of the dried coconut meat, called copra. The oil thus obtained is not initially suitable for human consumption. It must first be deodorized, bleached, and filtered.

In this method, high temperatures, bleaching agents, sodium hydroxides, and hot steam can be used to remove unwanted substances like the smoky flavor from the coconut oil. Unfortunately, these processes also largely destroy the oil's natural vitamins and antioxidants.

Coconut oil produced industrially is, despite the expensive and time-consuming process used to make it, much cheaper than organic virgin coconut oil. But don't let price sway you toward the cheaper product—it's just not worth it.

VIRGIN COCONUT OIL FATTY ACID PROFILE

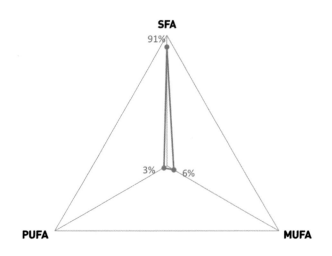

SFA = saturated fatty acids
PUFA = polyunsaturated fatty acids
MUFA = monounsaturated fatty acids

RECIPES

In these recipes, the coconut milk used is full-fat Thai Kitchen, in a tetra-pak (to avoid BPA). Fat-reduced coconut milk is not recommended, since the composition of macronutrients (protein, carbohydrates, and fats) in fat-reduced milk isn't balanced and doesn't fall into the Pure Food recommendations.

Look for good-quality organic coconut oil that's labelled "virgin." These varieties can be purchased in health food stores or ordered online. Again, cheap coconut oils are highly processed and should be avoided.

LOOK FOR GOOD-QUALITY ORGANIC COCONUT OIL THAT'S LABELED "VIRGIN."

ALTERNATIVES

If you do not like coconut milk and dairy products do not cause digestive problems for you, then you can replace coconut milk 1:1 with organic heavy cream in any of the recipes. Instead of coconut oil, you can use ghee or clarified butter, also 1:1.

Warning: Coconut flour is very absorbent and therefore it is *not* possible to simply replace it with another flour.

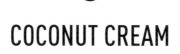

COCONUT CREAM

PREPARATION I

Put the coconut milk in the fridge for at least twenty-four hours before you use it.

Open the coconut milk without shaking the container. You want to avoid remixing the separated liquid water with the coconut cream, which will be on top of the container.

Scoop out the coconut cream with a spoon. You can use the remaining coconut water in the container for smoothies or drink it by itself.

Mix the coconut cream in a bowl with an electric mixer until it's airy and creamy.

.

PREPARATION II

Shake the coconut milk well. The milk should not be out of the fridge!
It should be very liquid and homogeneous.
Pour the coconut milk into a whipped cream dispenser, close the dispenser tightly.
Push one C02 cartridge into the dispenser according to the instruction.
Take the capsule off and shake the dispenser 5 to 10 times.
Then put the dispenser into the fridge for a few hours before using.

INGREDIENTS

2 cups (500 ml) coconut milk

COLORFUL COCONUT SMOOTHIES

Put all ingredients in a mixing bowl and mash with a hand blender
or in a food processor.

Immediately drink or bottle and bring it with you.

Instead of banana, use 5.2 oz (150 g) ripe mango.

COCONUT-BANANA | 1 SERVING

0.4 cups (100 ml) coconut milk
0.4 cups (100 ml) water
(or the corresponding amount of ice cubes)
1 banana
1 oz (30 g) instant organic gelatin
1 tsp (5 ml) ground cinnamon (optional)
1 tsp (5 ml) crushed turmeric (optional)
1 small pinch salt

COCONUT-BEET | 1 SERVING

*Use the same ingredients as in the
Coconut-Banana Smoothie, except:
½ banana (instead of a whole banana)
add 3.5 oz (100 g) beetroot, cooked*

COCONUT-BLUEBERRY | 1 SERVING

*Use the same ingredients as in the
Coconut-Banana Smoothie, except:
½ banana (instead of a whole banana)
add 3.5 oz (100 g) blueberries, fresh or frozen*

COCONUT KAISERSCHMARRN

(a pancake torn in pieces)

PREPARATION

Separate the eggs. In a bowl, mix the egg whites
with the salt until stiff.

In another bowl, mix well egg yolks, coconut milk, water,
gelatin/protein powder, and cinnamon with a hand mixer.
Sift the coconut flour over the mixture and blend in.

Mix in the stiff egg whites with a spoon.

Cook in three to four servings in a non-stick pan. Heat up a bit of coconut oil in a pan,
pour a quarter of the dough into the pan, and cook until little bubbles pop up
on the surface.

Now carefully turn the dough. It does not matter if it breaks.
Again, add a little coconut oil to the pan, so this side is also golden brown.
Shortly before the dough is cooked through (after about 10 minutes),
divide the dough into bite-sized pieces. Remove from pan and keep warm.
Repeat with the remaining dough.

SERVING SUGGESTIONS

Apple Schmarrn: Put the Kaiserschmarrn on plates and
top with peeled apple slices, then drizzle with a bit of honey.

Austrian: Serve with plum compote instead of apples.

American: Serve with fried bacon and maple syrup instead of apples.

Or simply serve with any kind of fruit.

8 eggs
0.8 cups (200 ml) coconut milk
0.8 cups (200 ml) water
2.8 oz (80 g) instant organic gelatin or neutral/vanilla
protein powder
1 tsp (5ml) cinnamon
2 pinches of salt
2.1 oz (60 g) coconut flour
4 tbsp (60 ml) liquid honey
14.1 oz (400 g) apples, peeled, cut into thin slices

3–4 SERVINGS

2 tbsp (30 ml) coconut oil

4 tbsp (60 ml) yellow curry powder

7 oz (200 g) bell peppers

7 oz (200 g) cauliflower

7 oz (200 g) sweet potatoes

1.3 cups (300 ml) water

1.3 lbs (600 g) prawns, cooked, peeled

1 cup (250 ml) full-fat coconut milk

1 tbsp (15 ml) fish sauce

salt

pepper

bunch fresh cilantro or basil leaves,
   plucked from the stem and washed

chili flakes (optional)

spring onions (optional)

PALEO CURRY

PREPARATION

Wash the vegetables, and chop them into similar-sized cubes
(about ½ in or 1.5 cm cubes).

Warm the coconut oil in a frying pan, add the curry paste, and fry briefly until the smell
of the curry rises. Add the vegetables and deglaze with water.
Simmer until the vegetables are cooked al dente (about 20 minutes).

Add prawns, coconut milk, and fish sauce and cook everything (don't boil!)
until the prawns are hot.

Add cilantro/basil and cook to taste. Season with salt and pepper.

SERVING SUGGESTIONS

Arrange on plates and enjoy immediately, or split portions into reusable containers.
You can reheat in the microwave or in a small pan (you may need to add a little water).
This will keep in the refrigerator for two or three days, or you can keep it in
the freezer for up to three months.

ALTERNATIVES

You can leave out the sweet potatoes and serve with cooked rice instead.
Note that rice contains more carbohydrates and is not ideal for losing weight.

Instead of prawns, you can use chicken breast, beef, pork, or veal.

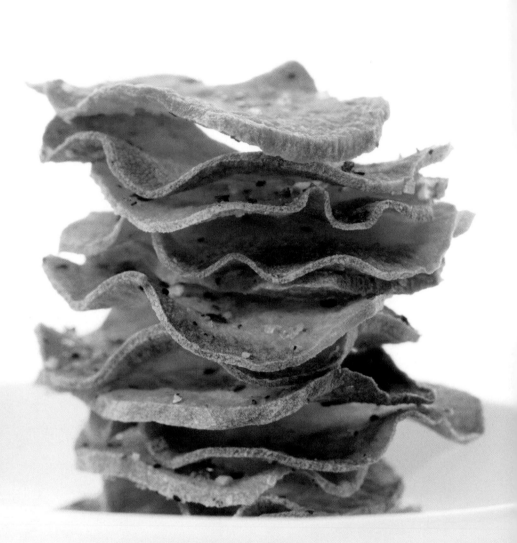

3–4 SERVINGS

10.5 oz (300 g) sweet potatoes
2 tbsp (30 ml) coconut oil
sea salt

COCONUT SWEET POTATO CHIPS

PREPARATION

Preheat the oven heat to 400°F (200°C). Line the baking tray with baking paper.

Peel the sweet potatoes and slice very thinly with a mandoline into approximately 2 mm thick slices.

In a bowl, melt the coconut oil.
Add the sweet potato slices in the dish and mix well until all the potato slices are coated with a layer of oil. This is best done with your hands.
Place the potato slices next to each other on the baking tray, using two baking sheets or baking the slices in portions.

Once the chips are brown at the edge, remove from the oven.
They will only really get crispy after they have cooled.

The exact baking time depends on the oven and the potatoes—just keep an eye on the chips and watch for the telltale brown edges.

SERVING SUGGESTIONS

Serve with guacamole or liver pâté.

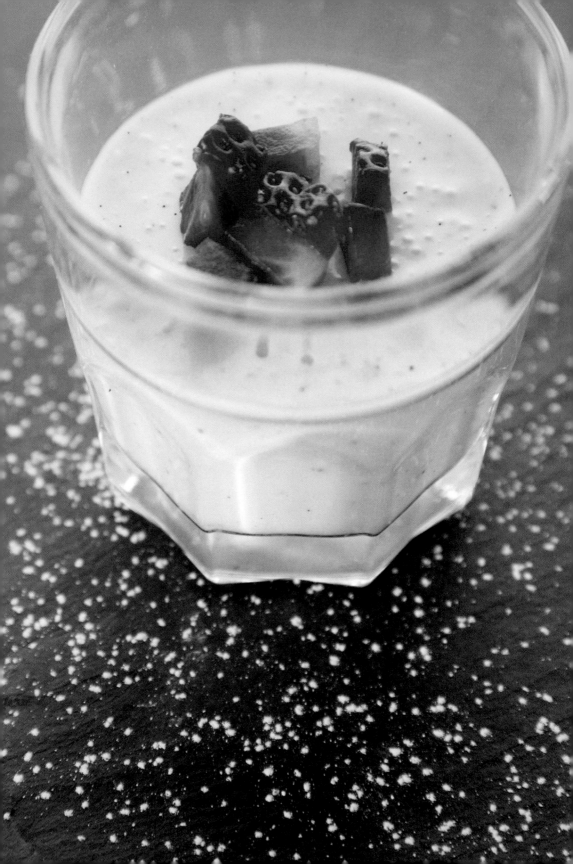

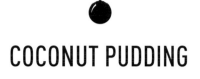

COCONUT PUDDING

PREPARATION

In a small bowl, soak the gelatin leaves in water.

In a big mixing bowl, place the coconut milk, instant gelatin/protein powder, sugar, and vanilla powder. Mix well with a hand blender.
(You can also mix the ingredients in a food processer.)

Remove the water from the soaked gelatin.
Add 2 tbsp (30 ml) of boiling water to the instant gelatin and stir until the gelatin has completely dissolved.

Add the dissolved gelatin into the big bowl, stirring constantly, and mix well.
Pour into small glasses and let chill for at least four hours in the refrigerator.

SERVIING SUGGESTIONS

Serve with fresh fruit and/or fruit sauce
(e.g., blueberries, mixed berries, peach, mango).
Melt chocolate (72 percent cocoa) and pour on the pudding.

3-4 DESSERT PORTIONS

2 gelatin leaves
enough water to soak the gelatin leaves according to the directions on your package
1 cup (250 ml) full fat coconut milk (e.g., Thai Kitchen)
1 oz (30 g) instant organic gelatin or neutral/vanilla protein powder
1 oz (30 g) powdered sugar or honey
1 tbsp (15 ml) Bourbon vanilla powder

COCONUT MACAROONS

Preheat the oven heat to 350°F (180°C). Line a tray with baking paper.

In a bowl, mix the egg whites with a pinch of salt until stiff.
Add the sugar in portions and mix until it has dissolved and a glossy,
rigid mass has formed.

Mix the grated coconut gently with a spatula into the rigid egg white–sugar mixture.

Divide the mixture into portions with two spoons to form clumps
and place on the baking tray.

Bake the macaroons 20 to 25 minutes,
until they're crisp and have turned golden brown on the outside.

When the macaroons are cooled, melt the chocolate in a small bowl.
Dip the bottom of each macaroon into the melted chocolate and put back on the
baking sheet. Wait until the chocolate is firm.

STORAGE

The coconut macaroons can be stored for about a week in an airtight tin.

FOR 15 PIECES

2 large egg whites
1 pinch of salt
1.4 oz (40 g) fine raw sugar
3.5 oz (100 g) grated coconut
1.7 oz (50 g) dark chocolate with at
    least 72 percent cocoa (optional)

4–8 SERVINGS

2 cups (500 ml) coconut milk
2 egg yolks
2 tsp (10 ml) ground cinnamon
1 oz (30 g) liquid honey

CINNAMON-COCONUT ICE CREAM

PREPARATION WITH AN ICE CREAM MAKER

Combine all ingredients in a blender, mix well, and then continue according
to the instructions of your ice cream maker.

Immediately enjoy or freeze.

PREPARATION WITHOUT AN ICE CREAM MAKER

Combine all ingredients in a blender and mix well.
Place in a shallow re-sealable container.

Place in the freezer for thirty minutes. Remove and mix well in the blender again.
Repeat this process about four times until the ice cream can no longer be mixed.
(All this mixing prevents the formation of ice crystals.)
After about four hours, the ice cream is ready to eat.

If you keep this in the freezer longer, you might need to take it out for
about 30 minutes before serving so that it softens enough.

SERVING SUGGESTIONS

Put a scoop of ice cream on a piece of brownie and garnish with
Coconut Cream and hot chocolate sauce.

VARIATIONS

Substitute vanilla powder or the contents of two scraped vanilla pods for the cinnamon.
Substitute gingerbread spices for the cinnamon, and serve with a gluten-free treat
or gingerbread.

OLIVE OIL

1. U.S. Extra-virgin Olive Oil
2. U.S. Virgin Olive Oil
3. U.S. Olive Oil

(There are a couple more grades that I won't even bother describing as they are so poor!) Note that these are voluntary grades, and that finding good-quality olive oil in the United States can be a challenge, though there is high-grade olive oil available to savvy consumers.

Virgin and extra-virgin olive oil are pure olive juice from the fruit harvest. The oil is extracted through mechanical means (pressure), without any chemical aids. Olive oil can be called "cold-pressed" when the temperature during the mechanical extraction never rises above 90°F (33°C); at higher temperatures, the nutrients and flavors evaporate. Good olive oil should have a slightly grassy flavor and taste fresh. Mild oil is very soft on the palate, average has pepper, tomato, banana, and almond notes. Intensive olive oil tastes strongly of olives and bitter almond.

Intensive olive oils are often a mix of different single-origin olive oils. Neutral oils are mixtures of three varieties, so that no flavor note becomes too strong.

The acidity of the oils also varies by grade. In virgin olive oil, the acidity must not exceed 0.8 percent—and the lower the acidity, the better. This information usually appears on the labels of olive oils.

The taste and quality also depend on how quickly the olives are pressed after the harvest.

BENEFITS OF OLIVE OIL OVER OTHER VEGETABLE OILS

In a nutshell: It keeps longer, and when heated, it goes through the fewest changes. Once oxygen, light, heat, or metals interact with other vegetable oils, the oils' fatty acids oxidize and decompose. If the oil is heated for cooking, the process proceeds even more quickly. The higher the unsaturated fatty acids in a vegetable oil, the more unstable and more prone to decomposition the oil is.

Virgin olive oil, however, is relatively stable. This is due to its high content of monounsaturated fatty acids. And it contains tocopherols, also known as Vitamin E, which further protect the olive oil from oxidation.

RECIPES

OLIVE OIL FATTY ACID PROFILE

In the following recipes, *only extra-virgin olive oil* is used, and it's never heated above 350°F (180°C), so that all its valuable elements are preserved. For roasting, I mostly use even more stable saturated fats like clarified butter, ghee, or coconut oil.

Warning: Never heat the oil over the smoking point—which you reach quickly if you're cooking marinated meat and fish.

Which olive oil you use is based on your personal preferences and what the dish you're making requires—but remember, make sure you have found a good source for unadulterated, extra-virgin olive oil no matter what blend you prefer.

When baking, a mild, more neutral oil works best.

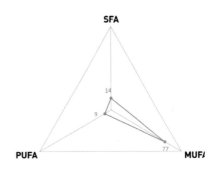

SFA = saturated fatty acids
PUFA = polyunsaturated fatty acids
MUFA = monounsaturated fatty acids

CHILI OLIVE OIL

5 dried red chilies
5 fresh red chilies
2 cups (500 ml) extra-
   virgin olive oil

ROSEMARY OLIVE OIL

5–10 sprigs fresh rosemary
2 cups (500 ml) extra-virgin
   olive oil

ORANGE-VANILLA OLIVE OIL

1 organic orange
1 vanilla pod
2 cups (500 ml) extra-virgin
   olive oil

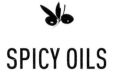

SPICY OILS

CHILI OLIVE OIL PREPARATION

Wash the fresh chilies and dry very well.
Place them and the dried chilies in a bottle and fill with olive oil.
Leave the bottle in a dark place for one to two weeks, then take the fresh chilies
from the bottle, so that the oil does not become cloudy.

ROSEMARY OLIVE OIL PREPARATION

Wash the rosemary and let it dry completely.
Place the rosemary stems in a clean, dry bottle, and fill it with olive oil.
Leave the bottle in a dark place for one to two weeks. Either consume relatively quickly
or decant the oil into a new bottle and remove the herbs.

ORANGE-VANILLA OLIVE OIL PREPARATION

Wash the orange and let it dry well.
Peel it with a vegetable peeler and add the peel and a vanilla bean and the oil to a bottle.
Seal the bottle well and store in a dark place at least two weeks.
Remove peel and vanilla bean.

SERVING SUGGESTIONS

Orange-Vanilla Olive Oil goes well with grilled fish fillet or
over cauliflower or exotic salad.

OLIVES IN PROSCIUTTO

PREPARATION

Cut the prosciutto in half lengthwise.
Wrap an olive in each length of prosciutto.
If necessary, fix in place with a toothpick.

SERVING SUGGESTIONS

These make great snacks or appetizers!

1–2 SNACK PORTIONS

10 black or green olives, pitted
6 slices lean prosciutto

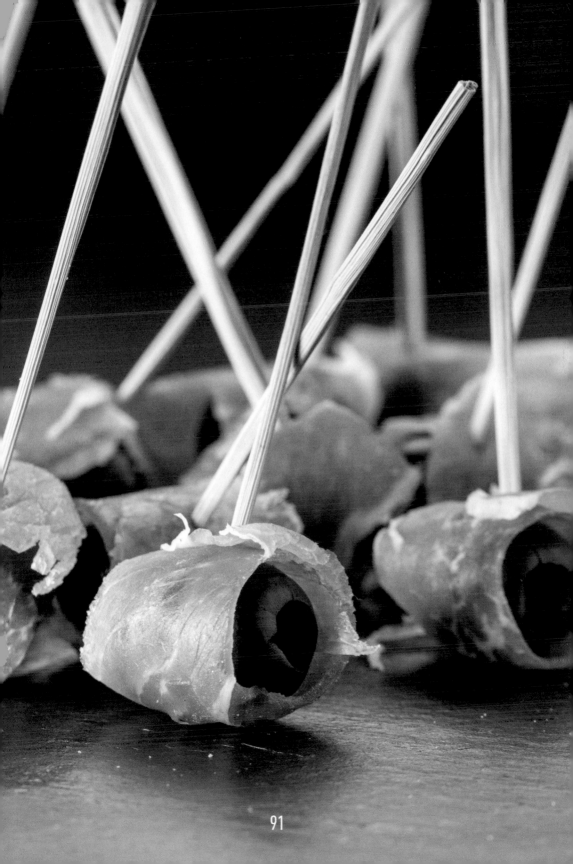

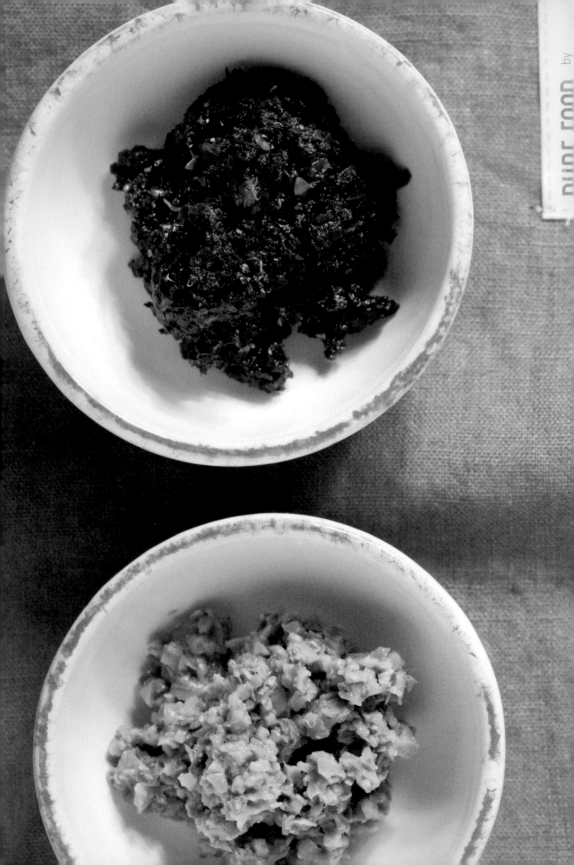

GREEN AND BLACK TAPENADE

PREPARATION

Add all ingredients except olive oil and pepper in a mixing bowl and mash with a hand blender, or combine in a food processor.

Slowly add the olive oil in portions until a thick paste is formed. Season with pepper.

SERVING SUGGESTIONS

Use to fill schnitzel rolls (recipe page 94–95).

Serve over steamed vegetables.

Serve over grilled lean meat, chicken breast, or fish fillet.

Easily diluted with olive oil as a sauce for rice noodles.

BLACK TAPENADE

3.5 oz (100 g) black olives, pitted
1 clove garlic, peeled
0.7 oz (20 g) capers
1.7 oz (50 g) olive oil
pepper

GREEN TAPENADE

3.5 oz (100 g) green olives, pitted
1 oz (30 g) anchovies, drained
0.7 oz (20 g) capers
1 tsp (5 ml) lemon juice
1 clove garlic, peeled
1.7 oz (50 g) olive oil
pepper

4 pork or turkey cutlets (each about 3.5 oz or 100 g)
4 servings green or black tapenade (about 1.7 oz or 50 g; recipe page 93)
1–2 tbsp (15–30 ml) clarified butter
1 tbsp (15 ml) tomato paste
1.3 lb (600 g) broccoli (or other seasonal vegetables)
1 tbsp (15 ml) olive oil
salt
pepper

SCHNITZEL ROLLS WITH TAPENADE FILLING

PREPARATION

Plate the schnitzel very thinly, then spread the tapenade on it and roll it up, securing the end of the roll with a toothpick.

Heat 1 tbsp (15 ml) of clarified butter in the frying pan and fry the schnitzel rolls on every side. Move to a gratin dish and place in the oven for about 20 minutes to finish cooking.

Boil the pan drippings in the frying pan with a little water and thicken with the tomato paste. Season with salt and pepper.

Wash the broccoli and cut it into equal-sized pieces.
Cook in the steamer or microwave until al dente.
After cooking, add salt, pepper, and 1 tbsp (15 ml) of olive oil.

SERVING SUGGESTIONS

Cover the rolls and the vegetables with the sauce.
Root puree (recipe page 97) would be a great addition here too!

SWEET POTATO OR POTATO PUREE

....

1.1 lbs (500 g) sweet potatoes or potatoes
2 tbsp (30 ml) olive oil
about 3.3 tbsp (50 ml) coconut oil or raw milk
1 tsp (5 ml) sea salt
1 tsp (5 ml) cinnamon (optional with sweet potatoes)
nutmeg, grated (optional with potatoes)

PARSNIPS OR PARSLEY ROOT PUREE

....

1.1 lbs (500 g) parsnip or parsley root
2 tbsp (30 ml) olive oil
about 3.3 tbsp (50 ml) coconut oil or raw milk
1 tsp (5 ml) sea salt
1 tsp (5 ml) ground coriander
1 tbsp (15 ml) gomasio (black, salted sesame seeds)

ROOT PUREES WITH OLIVE OIL

PREPARATION

Peel the root vegetables and cut into equal-sized pieces.
Boil in about 8 cups (2 liters) of well-salted water in a saucepan.
Cook the vegetables 15–30 minutes until soft. The cooking time will
vary depending on the type of vegetable and the size of the pieces.

Drain the vegetables in a colander.

Return the vegetable pieces to the pot.
Puree the liquid and vegetables with a hand blender.
Add more liquid if the puree isn't creamy enough.

Season with spices, herbs, and olive oil. If the puree is too thick, it
can be diluted slightly with broth, coconut milk, or heavy cream.

ALTERNATIVE

Instead of olive oil you can use coconut oil or butter.
Experiment with other herbs and spices.

SERVING SUGGESTIONS

Purees go well with grilled meat, fish, and poultry, Oriental Lamb
Stew (recipe page 150), Lamb Chops (recipe page 146), or Schnitzel
Rolls with Tapenade Filling (recipe page 94).

TIP

Cauliflower puree—a low-carb replacement
Prepare, wash, and cut the cauliflower into pieces. Cook in boiling
salted water until soft. Then continue as with the root puree.

10–12 PIECES

1.7 oz (50 g) defatted cocoa powder

½ cup (125 ml) boiling water

⅔ cup (150 ml) olive oil, mild

3 eggs

1.7 oz (50 g) of honey

1.7 oz (50 g) coconut flour

1 tsp (5 ml) baking soda

2 tsp (10 ml) vanilla sugar

1 pinch salt

OLIVE OIL CAKE

PREPARATION

Line a 9 in (23 cm) springform pan with baking paper
and brush the top with olive oil.

Put the cocoa powder into a bowl.
Gently add the boiling water in portions, stirring constantly until a creamy,
slightly liquid mass has formed. Allow to cool in the bowl.

Using a mixer, stir olive oil, eggs, and honey until a thick, airy,
fluffy cream has formed. Now slowly add the cocoa mixture to the cream.
Sift the coconut flour over the mixture,
then add the baking soda, vanilla sugar, and salt and mix again.
Pour the batter into the springform pan and spread evenly.

Bake 40–45 minutes, until the edges are firm and the middle of the cake
still looks slightly moist.

Allow to cool 10 minutes in the springform pan.
Loosen at the edge with a knife before removing the cake.

SERVING SUGGESTIONS

Enjoy while it's still hot or chill in the refrigerator for a few hours.

Serve with a scoop of ice cream.

Top with chocolate icing.

TIP

Cut the cake through the middle horizontally and thickly brush the center
with cold raw-milk butter, then reassemble into layers and enjoy.

NUTS

The selection of nuts and products made from them is vast. The less processed they are, the healthier. It's important that the nuts be fresh, not moldy, and raw if possible.

Mold is difficult to detect in its early stages. Therefore, only eat nuts whose expiration date has not passed and which have no rancid taste. Preferably, consume nuts unsalted and raw. Roasted and salted nuts are fine once in a while, but be warned that often nuts are roasted in vegetable oil.

Your nut consumption should be limited to a handful per day, as nuts contain a lot of simple and polyunsaturated fats. As mentioned earlier, our intake of omega-6 fatty acids needs to be reduced. A moderate consumption of nuts in combination with several saturated fats and plenty of omega-3 fatty acids is not a problem.

The various types of nuts differ greatly in their composition of macronutrients. The macadamia nut has the highest fat.

In these recipes I like to use organic walnuts, macadamia nuts, and pecans. Use any of those three nuts in these recipes.

Hazelnuts cause allergic reactions in many people and are moldy more often than other nuts. Cashews are seeds and cannot be eaten raw. They contain a lot of carbohydrates.

PEANUTS

Peanuts are not nuts. They belong to the legume family, and they often cause allergies. Also, the risk of mold in peanuts and peanut products (butter, for instance) is very high and occurs regularly. The composition of fatty acids in peanuts is not ideal—it has many polyunsaturated fatty acids.

SFA = *saturated fatty acids*
PUFA = *polyunsaturated fatty acids*
MUFA = *monounsaturated fatty acids*

FATTY ACID PROFILE OF VARIOUS NUTS

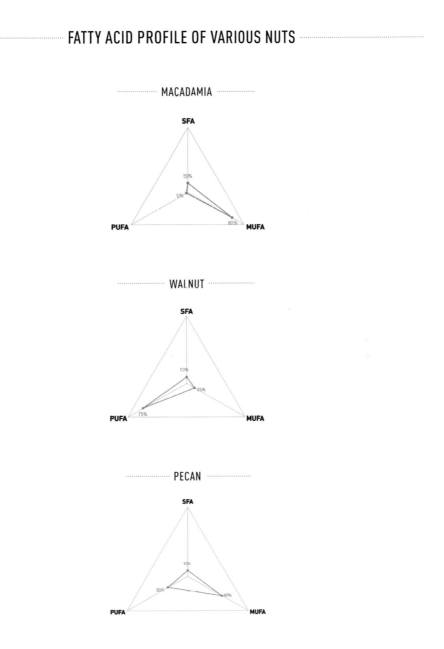

MACADAMIA

WALNUT

PECAN

NUT MUESLI

PREPARATION

Chop almonds and raisins in a food processor until almost a paste.

Chop walnuts coarsely and place in a large skillet.
Roast at medium-high heat until a nutty aroma rises and the nuts
are slightly brown.

Now add the pumpkin and sunflower seeds.

Reduce the heat to medium.

Roast the pumpkin seeds until they start to pop.
Spread the butter on the nuts and sprinkle in the raisin and
almond mixture. Season with cinnamon, ginger, and salt.

While the butter melts, keep stirring with a wooden spoon
and be careful that nothing burns.

After 3-5 minutes, when the nuts are light brown,
remove from the stove.

Now you can mix in the optional ingredients.
Once the muesli is cold, it is crispy and crunchy.

STORAGE

Sealed in an airtight container,
the muesli will keep up to two weeks.

NOTE

Muesli mixes alone are not balanced!
Always eat them with some protein too.

6-8 SERVINGS

1.7 oz (50 g) almonds
3.5 oz (100 g) raisins
3.5 oz (100 g) walnuts, coarsely chopped
1.7 oz (50 g) pumpkin seeds
1.7 oz (50 g) sunflower seeds
1:7 oz (50 g) butter
1 tsp (5 ml) ground cinnamon,
1 tsp (5 ml) ground ginger
1 pinch sea salt
1.7 oz (50 g) chia seeds (optional)
1.7 oz (50 g) whole flaxseed (optional)
1.7 oz (50 g) cocoa nibs (optional)

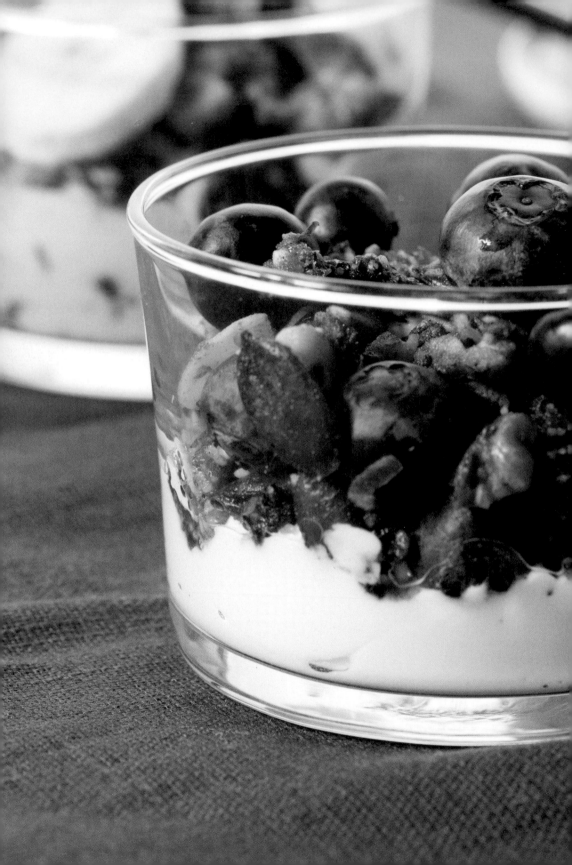

MUESLI WITH RAW MILK

2.1 oz (60 g) nut muesli mix
3.5 oz (100 g) raw-milk quark
0.4 cups (100 ml) raw milk
3.5 oz (100 g) berries

PREPARATION

Add the muesli to a bowl of quark and milk,
and sprinkle with berries.

MUESLI WITH COCONUT MILK

2.1 oz (60 g) nut muesli mix
0.7 oz (20 g) instant gelatin or egg white powder
3.3 tbsp (50 ml) coconut milk
3.3 tbsp (50 ml) water
1.7 oz (50 g) banana

PREPARATION

Puree gelatin or egg white powder, coconut
milk, water, and banana. Mix the puree with
the muesli in a bowl.

1.7 oz (50 g) chocolate (72 percent cocoa)
3.5 oz (100 g) walnuts, peeled
1 tsp (5 ml) cinnamon

CHOCOLATE-NUT BUTTER

PREPARATION

Break the chocolate into pieces and puree with walnuts and cinnamon in a food processor for 3–5 minutes until creamy.

STORAGE

Can be stored in a jar about two weeks. Do not refrigerate, as the butter will be too hard to spread.

SERVING SUGGESTIONS

Dessert: Spread 1 oz (30 g) of the Chocolate-Nut Butter on 3.5 oz (100 g) of apple or pear slices.

Recipe for a muesli: Mix 1.7 oz (50 g) Chocolate-Nut Butter, 7 oz (200 g) raw-milk quark, and a little apple, a banana or a small pear. Makes a meal.

3-4 SERVINGS

1.3 lbs (600 g) parsnips, sweet potatoes
   or other root vegetables
14.1 oz (400 g) cauliflower
14.1 oz (400 g) broccoli
1–2 tbsp (15–30 ml) olive oil
salt
pepper
1.3 lbs (600 g) fish fillet (e.g., trout)
3.5 oz (100 g) almonds, roasted, salted and ground
1 tsp (5 ml) salt, if nuts are not salted
2 eggs
0.7 oz (20 g) coconut flour
2 tbsp (30 ml) clarified butter

FISH IN NUT CRUST

PREPARATION

Wash, prepare, and cut the vegetables into bite-sized pieces.
Boil the root vegetables in salted water until tender.
Steam cauliflower and broccoli.

Put the vegetables in a bowl, add salt and pepper,
and pour in the olive oil.

Mix well so that all the vegetable pieces are seasoned and oiled.
In a soup bowl, lightly beat the eggs, sift the coconut flour into a second
dish, and place the minced nuts mixed with salt into a third dish.

Add the clarified butter to the pan and let it melt on medium heat.
Wash the fish fillets, pat dry, then press the fillets into the coconut
flour (both sides). Next, put them into the beaten eggs, let the excess
egg drip off, and press coated fillets into the minced nuts. Press on
the nuts well, so when you roast the fish a good crust will form.

SERVING SUGGESTIONS

Prepare only fish (smaller pieces) and serve as a snack or appetizer.

ALTERNATIVES

Instead of ground almonds, you can use macadamias or pecans.

The nut crust also works well with turkey cutlets
or chicken breast.

ABOUT 8 SERVINGS

1 bunch fresh basil, plucked from the stem and washed
5 cloves garlic, peeled
1.7 oz (50 g) pine nuts or other nuts
juice from ½–1 lemon
1.7 oz (50 g) Parmesan (optional)
3.3 tbsp (50 ml) olive oil
approximately 1 tsp (5 ml) salt
pepper

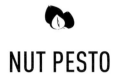

NUT PESTO

PREPARATION

Put all ingredients in a mixing bowl and puree with a hand blender
or in a food processor.

If you need to, add a little more olive oil and stir the puree with
a spoon until it has the right creamy consistency.
Season with salt and pepper.

STORAGE

Can be preserved in a storage jar in the refrigerator
for about two weeks.

SERVING SUGGESTIONS

Goes well with steamed vegetables, grilled meat,
chicken breast, or fish.

ASPARAGUS NOODLES WITH WALNUT PESTO

Cut fresh asparagus with a vegetable peeler into
strips/noodles.

Heat olive oil and walnut pesto in a frying pan.
Add the asparagus noodles, mix well, and sauté until
the noodles are nicely coated with the olive oil and pesto
and are still slightly crunchy.

This takes only a few minutes and makes a fine, tasty meal.

APPLE WITH NUT FILLING

PREPARATION

Preheat the oven to 350°F (180°C).

In a bowl, mix walnuts, butter, raisins, cinnamon,
and salt to a thick paste.

Wash, dry, and cut off the top third of the apples.

Remove the core from both halves, including stem.

Place the apple bottoms in a baking dish and fill with the nut paste.

Replace the cut-off ("lid") portions of the apples and bake for about
30 minutes. Remove from the oven, leave to cool for 5–10 minutes.

Remove the "lids" of the apples and add a dollop of Coconut Cream
on top. Then replace the "lids" once more.

SERVING SUGGESTIONS

Serve as a dessert after a protein-rich,
low-carbohydrate meal.
Replace Coconut Cream with about 8.8 oz (250 g) raw-milk quark
and serve as a main meal.

4 medium apples or pears (each about 4.5 oz or 130 g)
2.1 oz (60 g) walnuts, chopped (not ground!)
2.1 oz (60 g) butter, room temperature
1.4 oz (40 g) raisins, very finely chopped
1 tsp (5 ml) cinnamon
2 pinches salt
0.4 oz (100 ml) Coconut Cream (recipe page 70)

30 PIECES

2 eggs

3.5 oz (100 g) almonds, ground

1.7 oz (50 g) coconut fibers

1 tsp (5 ml) salt

2.6 oz (75 g) honey or finely ground raw sugar

3.5 oz (100 g) protein powder (neutral or vanilla; alternatively, use organic instant gelatin)

1.7 oz (50 g) whole almonds

1.7 oz (50 g) chocolate with at least 72 percent cocoa, finely diced (optional)

ALMOND-CHOCOLATE BISCOTTI

PREPARATION

In a bowl, beat the eggs well.
Combine all the ingredients except the almonds and chocolate cubes
and knead well.
The dough should be compact and slightly tacky.

Now add almonds and chocolate and knead into a roll
approximately 1.2 in (3 cm) in diameter.

Place in the refrigerator for 30 minutes.

Preheat the oven to 350°F (180°C). Line a tray with baking paper.

Remove the roll from the refrigerator and place on baking sheet.
Bake 30 minutes. Remove from the oven and allow to cool briefly.

Place the roll on a cutting board and carefully cut with
a sharp knife into 0.3 in (1 cm) slices.

Place the slices side by side on the baking sheet
and bake again until golden, 3–5 minutes.

STORAGE

Keep in an airtight tin for up to about two weeks.

SERVING SUGGESTIONS

1–2 pieces with espresso after dinner.

As a snack or once in a while for a sweet breakfast (with the protein
powder, the pastry is perfectly balanced in the composition of nutrients).

LARD

WHAT IS GOOD-QUALITY MEAT?

The following factors affect the meat quality positively:
- Species-appropriate feeding and farming
- Stress-free slaughter
- Short transportation to slaughter
- Careful processing of meat
- Adequate storing and curing time
- Clean facilities and processing

The meat color is a sign of good quality. Meat is often placed in commercial equipment with special lights that make it look pink and fresh. Ask to see the meat in daylight before you buy it.

Pork should be light to dark pink. White, watery pork tastes bland and comes from animals fattened too quickly (and then in cooking meat becomes dry and brittle). Suboptimal genetics (genetic predisposition) may be a reason.

Through breeding, pork meat has become much leaner, and most people cut off the visible fat of pork chops.

Pig products we prefer are fried bacon, pork belly, trotters, and pork chops with a fatty edge. These pieces contain more healthy fatty acids.

Lard is a pure, natural fat obtained by melting the back or kidney fat (subcutaneous fat) at 170°F to 215°F (80°C to 100°C). At room temperature, it is soft; stored in the refrigerator, it is solid. Unfortunately, this fat is not offered in supermarkets. It is ideal for roasting, frying, and for fine pastries.

PASTURED ORGANIC IS A MUST

Pork meat must be pastured organic because environmental toxins and residual antibiotics are stored in adipose tissue. To reduce your intake of these toxins, you have to choose organic, pastured meat. If you can not afford organic pork, it is better to eat lean pieces, roasted with clarified butter and refined with butter or olive oil.

DOES PORK CAUSE GOUT?

The trigger for gout is the substance purine. It can cause increased uric acid in the body, which may cause gout. Purine is a building block of genes and occurs everywhere—in meat and in plants. People with gout must be careful not just with meat consumption, but also with some plants, like beans.

LARD FATTY ACID PROFILE

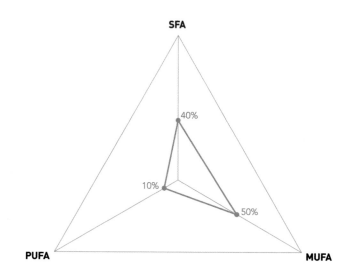

SFA

40%

10%

50%

PUFA

MUFA

SFA = saturated fatty acids
PUFA = polyunsaturated fatty acids
MUFA = monounsaturated fatty acids

We buy our pork at organic farms or from health food stores.
We love fried bacon and nicely marbled chops.

WHAT TO KNOW WHEN YOU'RE BUYING MEAT
(THIS APPLIES TO ALL MEAT, FISH, AND POULTRY GRADES)

- Read the label and pay attention to the price. Vacuum-packed meat is often imported and of poor quality.
- High-quality meat shines and is dry. Meat soaked in its own juice can be spoiled.
- Good meat has a more solid consistency. Test it with your finger—the imprint should bounce back and not linger.
- Check the meat color! Graying is an indication that the meat isn't good anymore.
- Do not buy pre-marinated meat. It is difficult to see if the meat is fresh, and they may use gluten-containing spice mixes.
- Good meat smells neutral to slightly acidic.

3-4 SERVINGS

4 eggs

0.4 cup (100 ml) coconut milk or raw milk

1 tsp (5 ml) salt

1 tsp (5 ml) apple cider vinegar (optional)

1 oz (30 g) coconut flour

2.8 oz (80 g) cassava or tapioca flour (gluten-free)

20 strips fried bacon

1.3 lbs (600 g) cherry or grape tomatoes

onions, peeled and finely chopped, to taste (optional)

butter for ramekins or refractory espresso cups

FRIED BACON WITH POPOVERS

Preheat the oven to 425°F (220°C).
Grease ramekins or refractory espresso cups with butter.

In a bowl, use a hand blender to combine 2 whole eggs and 2 yolks,
coconut milk, salt, and apple cider vinegar (you can also use
a food processor). You can use a blender or a mixer.
Sift coconut flour and cassava or tapioca flour over the dough and mix well.

In a separate bowl, beat 2 egg whites until stiff.
Add the stiff egg whites gently to the egg-milk-flour mixture.

Spread the batter into the cups or ramekins and bake for
20 minutes in the oven.

Meanwhile, fry the bacon in a skillet over medium heat until crispy.
Remove the bacon from the pan and keep warm.

In the pan, fry the tomato and onion in the bacon fat until soft.

Remove the popovers from the oven and let cool slightly. Remove from
the cups and serve with the fried bacon and tomatoes.

ALTERNATIVES

Serve the popovers with soup.

Spread the popovers with butter and a little honey.

Make a popover sandwich: cut the cold popovers in the middle, spread
with butter, and fill with cold meat or unpasteurized cheese.

RICE NOODLES WITH CARBONARA SAUCE

PREPARATION

Boil 8 cups (2 liters) of water with 1 tsp (5 ml) salt and cook the rice noodles until just tender according to instructions on the package.

In a frying pan, fry pancetta or bacon until crispy.

Add the rice noodles to the pan. If necessary add a little olive oil, and fry 1–2 minutes. In a large serving bowl, whisk eggs and yolks together, season with pepper, and stir in half the grated cheese.

Empty the entire contents of the pan into the bowl with the egg-cheese mixture just before serving. Mix well and enjoy immediately.

NOTE

Never empty the egg-cheese mixture into the hot pan; you'll get scrambled eggs instead of a liquidy, creamy carbonara sauce.

SERVING SUGGESTIONS

Sprinkle the dish with the remaining cheese and season with pepper.

Serve with a large green salad or steamed spinach.

VARIATIONS

Instead of rice noodles, use zucchini noodles
Cut 7–10.5 oz (200–300 g) of zucchini into thin strips, add to the pancetta/bacon pan, and fry for a few minutes.

Sweet potato noodles
Cut 5.2–7 oz (150–200 g) peeled sweet potatoes into thin (2 mm) strips, blanch for 2–3 minutes in boiling salted water, then add to the pan with the pancetta or bacon and fry briefly.

3-4 SERVINGS

7 oz (200 g) rice noodles, uncooked
1 tsp (5 ml) salt
3.5 oz (100 g) fried pancetta or bacon, cut into strips or cubes
1–2 tbsp (15–30 ml) olive oil
2 eggs
2 egg yolks
2.8 oz (80 g) Parmesan, Sbrinz or pecorino, freshly grated
salt
pepper

3-4 SERVINGS

3 tbsp (45 ml) tamari sauce (gluten-free)
1 tbsp (15 ml) sambal oelek
1 tbsp (15 ml) honey
1 oz (30 g) ginger, freshly grated
2 spring onions, sliced into rings
4 pork belly sections (each about 7 oz or 200 g)
2.2 lbs (1 kg) vegetables, prepared (e.g., pumpkin,
   sweet potatoes, potatoes, parsnips, etc.)
sea salt

MARINATED PORK BELLY

PREPARATION

Preheat the oven heat to 350°F (180°C). Line a tray with baking paper.
In a shallow dish, add tamari sauce, sambal oelek, honey, ginger,
and spring onions and mix well.

Cover the pork belly with marinade.
Marinate the pork belly for at least two hours, or overnight.
Be sure to turn at least once to ensure the marinade fully covers the meat.

Cut the vegetables into chunks of at least 0.6 inches (1.5 cm).
Place them onto the baking paper and add salt.

Lay the pork belly slices on the vegetables, so the fat
that emerges during baking can run over the vegetables.
Pour the remaining marinade over the vegetables.

Put the baking sheet in the oven.

After 20 minutes turn on the broiler to medium-high
and cook for another 10 minutes.

Take the tray out, turn the vegetables in the fat, and turn the pork belly slices
over and cook for another 5–10 minutes, taking care not to burn anything.

SERVING SUGGESTIONS

Serve with baked potatoes or sweet potatoes if these are not already
in your dish, or root vegetable puree.

In summer, a big green salad goes perfectly with the crispy pork belly.

3-4 SERVINGS

2 tbsp (30 ml) sesame oil
2 tsp (10 ml) sambal oelek
approximately 0.4 cup (100 ml) vegetable stock, hot
0.7 oz (20 g) honey or brown raw sugar
0.7 oz (20 g) fresh ginger, grated
1 lemon, juice and grated zest
14.1 oz (400 g) white cabbage
7 oz (200 g) carrots, peeled
7 oz (200 g) sweet apples
1 tbsp (15 ml) clarified butter
4 pork chops with bones (each about 7 oz or 200 g)
salt
pepper
1 tbsp (15 ml) butter
salt
cayenne pepper or pepper
2 spring onions, prepared and cut into fine strips
fresh cilantro, leaves picked from the stems

PORK CHOPS WITH ASIAN SALAD

PREPARATION

In a large salad bowl, mix the listed ingredients up to and including the lemon juice and zest to create the dressing.

Cut the cabbage into thin strips, grate the carrots and apples coarsely, and mix everything in the bowl with salad dressing.

Mix well and refrigerate.

Heat 1 tbsp (15 ml) clarified butter in a frying pan on medium-high, add salt and pepper to the chops on both sides, and place in the pan (possibly in portions if the pan does not have enough space!). Once drops of blood appear on top of the chops, turn over and continue to fry for 2–3 minutes.

Reduce the heat and add more butter to the pan.

Once the butter has melted, turn the chops again and drizzle with the melted butter.

Take the salad out of the fridge, again stir well, and season to taste with salt and cayenne pepper or black pepper.

SERVING SUGGESTIONS

Garnish the salad with onion slices, cilantro, and sesame seeds.

3–4 SERVINGS

1.1 lbs (500 g) sweet potatoes, peeled and cut into pieces
salt
pepper
1 tbsp (15 ml) butter
8 pork cutlets (each about 2.4 oz or 70 g)
4 slices cooked ham
2.8 oz (80 g) raw-milk cheese (e.g., Gruyère), cut into 4 slices
2 tbsp (30 ml) clarified butter
1.3 lbs (600 g) cucumber, already peeled and seeded
2 tbsp olive oil
1 bunch fresh dill, washed, leaves picked from the stems

UNBREADED CORDON BLEU

PREPARATION

Cook the sweet potatoes until tender in steamer or microwave.
Place in a gratin dish, add salt and pepper, and sprinkle with flakes of butter.
Bake at 350°F (180°C) for about 20 minutes, turning occasionally.

Flatten the meat so it becomes thinner and wider. Wrap a slice of ham around
a slice of cheese and place on one of the cutlets. Cover with another cutlet.
Use toothpicks to hold the side edges together, so that a little cheese can
run out from the Cordon Bleu.

Slice the cucumber and place in a salad bowl.
Add olive oil, dill, salt, and pepper and stir.

In a frying pan on medium-high heat, warm the clarified butter
and fry the Cordon Bleu. It takes about 4 minutes on each side.

SERVING SUGGESTIONS

Serve with sweet potatoes and a hearty salad on a separate plate.
This will keep in a refrigerator for three to four days.

VARIATIONS

Instead of sweet potatoes, serve with a puree of root vegetables.

BEEF FAT

QUALITY

As with all the other meat discussed, we recommend eating grass-fed, grass-finished (i.e., not fattened up on grains just before slaughter), pastured, organic beef whenever possible. It's better for the animal, for the planet, and for you. Grass-fed organic pastured meat is rich and tasty. It also has a much better fatty acid composition than grain-fed animals do. The fatty acid composition of conventionally raised cattle is not healthy.

From 1998 to 2009, the number of grass-fed beef producers in the United States grew from just 100 to over 2000, and now many if not most supermarkets have grass-fed meet available. Of course, buy your beef from farmers you know whenever possible, and consider entering an animal share—freeze a quarter or half of a cow in your deep freezer every year.

BEEF FAT FATTY ACID PROFILE

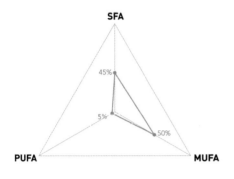

SFA = saturated fatty acids
PUFA = polyunsaturated fatty acids
MUFA = monounsaturated fatty acids

Humane husbandry and feeding are very important for the quality and nutritional value of beef.

Meat from cattle that has been fed with grains has a different fatty acid composition than grassfed beef.

RECIPES

We buy beef mostly in larger quantities directly from the farm. Pieces of meat that we won't eat immediately go in the freezer. We mainly eat the fattier cuts and offal. So per pound, the price for this very nutritious meat isn't too high. Pasture beef has another advantage: Due to the high nutrient content, the meat pieces can be somewhat smaller and you'll still be ingesting a lot of nutrients. Despite the smaller pieces/portions, we get more nutrients (healthy fatty acids, vitamins, and minerals) out of high-quality beef than from a larger piece of meat from a conventionally raised animal.

Pastured beef is often leaner than conventional meat because the animals are not fed grains. Tougher pieces need more time to cook so that the animal fibers soften—take this longer cooking time into consideration when you're meal planning. If you're cooking meat quickly, it helps if you marinate it with olive oil and spices and herbs. The result will be much better and softer.

MEAT FROM THE FREEZER
(APPLIES TO ALL MEAT, FISH, AND POULTRY VARIETIES)

Nutritionally and taste-wise, there's no reason not to use meat from the freezer.

TIPS FOR BUYING MEAT FROM THE FREEZER

- Don't buy any meat with freezer burn. Usually you find freezer burn on badly sealed packaging and/or gray spots in the border of the meat. Freezer burn occurs mostly when the freezing is disrupted during the transportation of the meat.
- Buy snow-free packaging. Ice crystals indicate that juice has left the meat—probably also due to too-warm temperatures. As a result, the meat is dry and soft after thawing. If you can't see the meat through the packaging, then try the shake test: If you hear crackling inside the package when you shake it, put it back!
- Slowly thaw the meat in the fridge.
- Thawed meat spoils faster than fresh. Therefore, we recommend a fast processing.
- Thawed meat should not be refrozen, otherwise there may be a significant loss of quality.

FREEZING MEAT YOURSELF

If you're planning to freeze meat yourself, observe the following guidelines:

- Lean meat can be stored longer than fatty cuts.
- Choose freezer bags or containers to freeze the meat; it will keep the quality of the meat better than inadequate wrapping.
- It's best to freeze meat as quickly as possible to avoid bacteria developing. It's therefore advisable to freeze meat in small portions so that it freezes through quickly and evenly.

TENDER GRASS-FED BEEF

To keep the meat tender and juicy:

- Rub both sides of the meat with sea salt (1 tsp or 5 ml for a 1 in or 2.5 cm thick steak).
- Put the meat into the fridge (1 hour for a 1 in or 2.5 cm thick steak, less than an hour for thinner pieces).
- Take it out of the fridge and wash the salt off with cold water.
- Pat the meat dry thoroughly.
- Grill or fry the meat.
- Season with pepper and a piece of butter.

This method can be used for all meats (beef, pork, calf, game, etc.).

COOKING LEVELS

Doneness of meat:

Level 1   Blue rare: thin, brown crust, inside almost raw and still bloody.
Level 2   Rare: crispy, brown crust, bloody core.
Level 3   Medium-rare: brown crust, inside pink throughout.
Level 4   Medium: meat inside should be only slightly pink.
Level 5   Very well done: no longer pink and completely cooked through.

4 beef bones, sliced, with marrow
sea salt

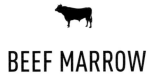

BEEF MARROW

PREPARATION

Fill a sealable container with cold water and soak the bones in it, in a refrigerator, for 24 hours. The bones must be completely covered with water.

Preheat the oven heat to 350°F (180°C).

Take the bones out of the water, rinse with cold water, pat dry, and lay side by side on a baking sheet or in a gratin dish.

Sprinkle sea salt on the marrow and roast the bones in the oven for 30 minutes.

SERVING SUGGESTIONS

Serve with a lean piece of meat and roasted vegetables.

The vegetables can be roasted along with the bone and will cook perfectly in the fat released from the bones.

MERGUEZ (NORTH AFRICAN SAUSAGES)

PREPARATION

In a bowl, mix well all ingredients up to and including the pepper.
Leave covered in the refrigerator for approximately 2 hours.

Divide the meat mixture into 12 sausages.
Place the sausages on the grill or in a hot pan and cook for 4–6 minutes.

Gently turn the sausages and cook for a further 4–6 minutes.

SERVING SUGGESTIONS

Serve immediately with salad and a wedge of lemon. Goes well with root puree.
You can make smaller sausages as an appetizer and dip in guacamole
(recipe page 56).

VARIATIONS

Replace the beef with lamb or use half beef, half lamb.

3-4 SERVINGS

1.1 lbs (500 g) minced beef (not lean)
1 tbsp (15 ml) sambal oelek or harissa
4 cloves garlic
1 tsp (5 ml) ground cumin
1 tsp (5 ml) fennel seeds, crushed or ground in a mortar
1 tsp (5 ml) sea salt
1 tsp (5 ml) black pepper
1 tsp (5 ml) cayenne pepper (optional)
1 lemon, quartered

3–4 SERVINGS

4 slices veal shank
  (per 7 oz or 200 g of bone)
1.4 oz (40 g) fresh ginger, peeled
2 stalks lemon grass
4 Kaffir lime leaves (optional)
2 small red chilies
1 tbsp (15 ml) fish sauce
4 pinches each salt and pepper
14.1 oz (400 g) carrots, peeled, halved
7 oz (200 g) celery, peeled,
  cut into 4 pieces
4 scallions
bunch of fresh chives
about 1.7 cups (400 ml) water

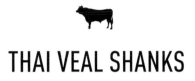

THAI VEAL SHANKS

Put all ingredients in a Dutch oven.
Fill with water until veal shanks are half submerged.

After it reaches a boil, reduce heat and simmer for 2 hours.

The meat is done when it's falling off the bone.

SERVING SUGGESTIONS

Serve a shank with roasted veggies and/or root puree.

VARIATIONS

Replace beef with lamb or use half beef, half lamb.

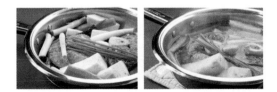

DIY BEEF TARTARE

PREPARATION

Get tartare fresh from your butcher,
or slice it very finely yourself at home just before serving.

Cut the meat into four portions and place on four plates.
It looks beautiful when you use a ring mold;
you can also layer the meat in a small bowl.

Push a space into the top of the meat and slip the yolks in carefully.

Place capers, pickles, shallots, etc., in small bowls on the table.
Also leave mustard and sauces out, so that everyone can prepare their
tartare to their personal taste.

SERVING SUGGESTIONS

Very good with lettuce, steamed vegetables, potatoes,
or Coconut Sweet Potato Chips (recipe page 78).

3–4 SERVINGS

1.3 lbs (600 g) beef fillet
4 egg yolks
4 tbsp (60 ml) capers, finely chopped
8 pickles, finely chopped
2 shallots, peeled and finely chopped
4 tbsp (60 ml) Dijon mustard
4 tbsp (60 ml) tamari sauce
4 tsp (20 ml) olive oil (optional)
1 bunch parsley, washed and finely chopped
Tabasco (optional)
salt
pepper

LIVER SALTIMBOCCA WITH BUTTERNUT SQUASH

PREPARATION

Preheat the oven heat to 350°F (180°C).
Grease a baking sheet with 1 tsp (5 ml) butter and place in the oven.

Cut the butternut squash into 8 pieces about 0.4 in (1 cm) thick. If the squash is small and elongated, you can cut more slices.

Remove the baking sheet from the oven and carefully lay the squash slices next to each other. Put some butter on the squash slices and add salt and pepper.
Bake for 20–25 minutes.

Wash the veal liver well under cold water and pat dry. Cut the liver transversely into 24 strips. Halve the bacon strip in the middle.

Each piece of liver should have a piece of bacon and a fresh sage leaf fixed with a toothpick—insert it so that the saltimbocca is nice and flat.

After the frying pan is hot, place the saltimbocca bacon side down in the pan. Reduce the heat and wait until the fat emerges from the bacon. Once the bacon is lightly browned and enough grease has leaked into the pan, turn the saltimbocca and finish cooking on the liver side.

Wash and spin dry the mâche. Peel the figs and cut into small cubes.

In a salad bowl mix well olive oil, balsamic vinegar, and figs, then season with salt and pepper. Mix in the mâche just before serving.

SERVING SUGGESTIONS

Arrange the squash slices on warmed plates.
Place the saltimbocca on the slices and sprinkle with fig balsamic.
Serve the mâche on the same plate.

ALTERNATIVE

Instead of veal liver, use beef or pork liver.

3-4 SERVINGS

14.1 oz (400 g) veal liver
12 strips fried bacon
24 fresh sage leaves
4 tsp (20 ml) fig balsamic vinegar
14.1 oz (400 g) butternut squash, peeled
2 tbsp (30 ml) butter
14.1 oz (400 g) mâche, washed and spun dry
2-3 tbsp (30-45 ml) olive oil
2 tbsp (30 ml) fig balsamic for garnish
4 small fresh figs
salt
pepper

LAMB FAT

The flavor of lamb is particularly dependent on what the animal is fed. Meat from livestock that is fed with grains contains a high concentration of omega-6 fatty acids. The taste is quite different from pastured lambs, whose meat also has higher levels of omega-3 fatty acids. These make the meat spicier and healthier.

Grass-fed lamb contains healthy fatty acids and many important minerals, especially iron, zinc, and niacin, which is important for cell and blood formation, strengthening the body's defenses, energy, and nervous system. In addition, lamb meat contains the vitamins A, C, D, K, and the B group, which are important for bone health and optimal metabolism.

L-CARNITINE

Lamb has up to 190 mg of L-carnitine per 100 grams, making it one of the best sources of this important amino acid. This compound is much better absorbed from food than it is from supplements. In the longer term, increased supply of L-carnitine in combination with exercise supports fat burning and also shows a number of positive effects, such as the vasodilator effect and strengthening the immune system.

WHEN IS A LAMB A SHEEP?

Lamb is the meat of animals slaughtered between their third and sixth month. It is bright pink, slightly streaked with fat, tender, and fine grained. Even more delicate is the meat of suckling lambs slaughtered between the fifth and eighth week of life.

The more species-appropriate and humane the sheep farming, the better the quality of meat.

LAMB FAT FATTY ACID PROFILE

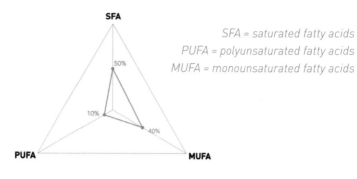

SFA = saturated fatty acids
PUFA = polyunsaturated fatty acids
MUFA = monounsaturated fatty acids

RECIPES

COOKING TIPS FOR LAMB

The meat should always be cut against the fiber direction, so you end up with short, tender meat fibers. The fatty edges should be kept on the meat. You can cut the fatty edges a few times so that the meat doesn't curl up during cooking. You can flatten lamb steaks and chops a bit by pressing them down with your palm.

If you plan to grill your lamb, salt it only after you turn it to cook the second side. Lamb, which has a very short cooking time, is best salted right before serving. Brown the meat first, then reduce the heat and slowly cook until done. But don't fry or cook it too long, because the lamb could lose flavor. The best flavor develops when the meat is still slightly pink in the center. Piercing or cutting the meat during preparation can dry it out and make it quite tough.

Lamb chops are our absolute favorite, especially grilled. Weekdays when we don't have much time, we place the cut chops on the grill for a few minutes and have a mixed salad to create a fast, nutrient-rich meal. On weekends, we prefer the whole rack of lamb. We leave it for 20–30 minutes on the grill so that the meat inside is still pink. Since we prefer the fatty cuts of meat, we only buy pastured or organic lamb.

3-4 SERVINGS

10 lamb chops (about 1 rack of lamb,
    approx. 25.5 oz or 700 g)
2 tbsp (30 ml) mustard
sea salt
pepper
1 tbsp (15 ml) clarified butter
fresh rosemary sprigs

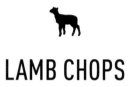

LAMB CHOPS

PREPARATION IN FRYING PAN

Rub the lamb chops on both sides with mustard, salt, and pepper.

Heat clarified butter with the rosemary sprigs in a frying pan over medium heat. Place the chops in the liquid clarified butter and fry 2–4 minutes per side to desired degree of doneness.

PREPARATION ON THE GRILL

Rub the lamb chops on both sides with mustard, salt, and pepper and grill.

TIP

Caveman-style dining
Eat the lamb chop right off the bone, holding it with your fingers.
Eat everything you can, including fat and tougher fibers from the bone.

about 15 stalks fresh rosemary
5 cloves garlic, finely chopped (optional)
0.4 cup (100 ml) olive oil
1 tsp (5 ml) pepper
1-2 tsp (5-10 ml) sea salt
1 leg of lamb, about 3.5 lbs (1.6 kg)
about 3.2 ft (1 m) string
about 2.6 lbs (1.2 kg) sweet potatoes
and/or root vegetables
1 tsp (5 ml) sea salt

LEG OF LAMB WITH SWEET POTATOES

PREPARATION

Preheat the oven heat to 400°F (200°C). Line a tray with baking paper.

For the marinade, wash 5 stalks rosemary and pat dry.
Pluck the green leaves and chop finely. Peel the garlic and chop finely.

In a small bowl, mix rosemary, garlic, olive oil, pepper, and salt.

Rinse the leg of lamb under cold water, pat dry, and tie the string around it
(as shown in image).

Put the 10 remaining rosemary stalks under the string on the fatty side of the
lamb leg. Brush the whole lamb leg with the marinade.

Place the marinated meat on the baking sheet and roast for 30 minutes in the oven.

Cut the sweet potatoes and/or vegetables into large equal pieces.

After 30 minutes, turn the heat down to 325°F (160°C).
Turn the lamb shank and add sweet potatoes and/or vegetables to the baking sheet.

After 1 hour rotate the lamb (the rosemary stalks will now be back on top).
Mix the sweet potatoes/vegetables in fat so that they are well oiled.

After a total of 2.5 hours, the meat should be tender inside, almost falling off
the bone, and have a crispy crust on the outside.

Take the leg out of the oven, cover, and let sit for 15 minutes to allow the meat
juices to soak into the flesh and not leak too much when you're cutting.

SERVING SUGGESTIONS

Keep sweet potatoes and vegetables warm in the oven till just before you serve
and add salt and pepper to taste.

1 onion
1.1 lbs (500 g) lamb
  shoulder, cut into pieces
2 tbsp (30 ml) clarified butter
1 tsp (5 ml) cinnamon
1 tsp (5 ml) paprika
1 tsp (5 ml) ground cumin
4.2 cups (1 liter) vegetable bouillon
10 dates, dried, de-stoned
1 oz (30 g) raisins
1.1 lbs (500 g) carrots, peeled and quartered
2 tbsp (30 ml) tomato puree or paste
salt
pepper
2 tbsp (30 ml) toasted flaked almonds

ORIENTAL LAMB STEW

PREPARATION

Peel and dice the onion.

Brown the lamb in hot clarified butter.

Add onions, cinnamon, paprika, and cumin and cook briefly.
Deglaze with vegetable broth, cover, and simmer for 1 hour at medium heat.
Add carrots, dates, and raisins to the stew and simmer another 30 minutes.
Thicken the sauce with the tomato puree, and season with salt and pepper.

SERVING SUGGESTIONS

Arrange the stew into soup bowls and sprinkle with flaked almonds.

For more sharpness, add some cayenne pepper.

For a sweeter taste, sprinkle a little cinnamon.

3-4 SERVINGS

7 oz (200 g) cucumber, peeled and seeded
3.5 oz (100 g) raw milk full-fat quark
1 tsp (5 ml) lemon juice
1 tbsp (15 ml) olive oil
sea salt
pepper
bunch of thyme
bunch of parsley
bunch of peppermint (optional)
14.1 oz (400 g) minced lamb
1 clove garlic, peeled and finely chopped
1 tsp (5 ml) sea salt
1 tsp (5 ml) pepper
8 strips fried bacon
2.1 oz (60 g) raw-milk feta cheese, sliced (optional)
4-8 large lettuce leaves or 7 oz (200 g) of lettuce
1.4 oz (40 g) watercress or sprouts
 avocado

SIGNATURE LAMB BURGER WITH TZATZIKI

PREPARATION

To make the tzatziki, grate the cucumber coarsely.
Mix it in a bowl with quark, lemon juice, olive oil, sea salt, and pepper.
Let it sit in the refrigerator for at least half an hour.

Wash, dry, and very finely chop all herbs. Add the minced lamb in a bowl
and knead with herbs, garlic, sea salt, and pepper.

Make three or four patties from the minced meat mixture.
Push a slight depression in the middle of each one with the palm of your hand
so that the patties will fry evenly.

Fry the bacon in a skillet until crispy. Remove and keep warm.
Fry the patties in the remaining bacon fat.

Divide the feta cheese into three or four servings.

Stir the tzatziki well before serving, and, if necessary,
add a little more salt and/or pepper.

SERVING SUGGESTIONS

Serve the burger tower (pictured) with lettuce and avocado as well as a fruit
for dessert for a fine, well-balanced meal.

POULTRY FAT

Ideally, our chickens would be roaming free across meadows, eating insects, worms, larvae, seeds, grains, and grasses. In practice, chickens are mostly industrially raised and processed, fed on just grains and soy, making them high in omega-6 fatty acids. It is possible to find good meat—usually the best approach is to find a farmer you trust, and even check out their farm in person if possible. If that's not possible for you, then carefully read the labels in the grocery story. The USDA's Agricultural Marketing Service is the authority on poultry labelling in the United States, and the label you want to watch for when you're seeking high-quality chicken is "Certified Organic."

Certified organic chicken comes from animals raised without antibiotics, hormones, genetic engineering, and artificial ingredients. Certified organic animals are allowed to move for exercise and must have species-appropriate stress reduction.

Note that other labels, such as "Free Range," "No Hormones," and "Naturally Raised," don't guarantee good meat quality or humanely raised animals. To be "Free Range," for example, chickens must have continuous access to the outdoors throughout their entire life cycle. And although free-range chickens might be out foraging for their food in a pasture all day, they may also be in a barn with hundreds or thousands of other chickens, with one door to the outside (which they may or may not ever use, and which may or may not lead to an idyllic pasture). Free range does not guarantee that the meat is free of hormones and antibiotics.

POULTRY FAT FATTY ACID PROFILE

CHICKEN

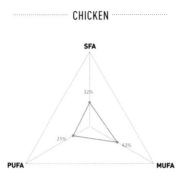

TURKEY

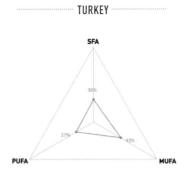

SFA = saturated fatty acids
PUFA = polyunsaturated fatty acids
MUFA = monounsaturated fatty acids

RECIPES

In these recipes I use only organic chicken. Never buy marinated poultry; the marinades include flavor enhancers, sugar, lactose, and starch flour (often at least partly with gluten).

You can eat the skin of organic hens, no problem. With conventionally raised chickens it's best to remove the skin; adipose tissue contains more toxins. Poultry should always be rinsed under cold water and patted dry with paper towels. All kitchen utensils that come into contact with raw poultry meat must be washed immediately with soap. Hands should be washed with soap after each contact with raw poultry meat so that no bacteria can be transmitted. Once poultry meat is cooked, the bacteria is rendered harmless.

> You can do a simple check with a wooden skewer to see whether a chicken breast or a whole chicken is cooked through: Put the skewer into the thickest part of the chicken breast. If the juice coming out of the breast is clear, then the chicken is cooked through. If the juice is still reddish (i.e., bloody), then the chicken needs longer to cook. This technique can be applied to any type of poultry.

All recipes can be cooked with different types of poultry—chicken, pheasant, turkey, etc.

6–8 SERVINGS

4 carrots
1 small celeriac
1 leek
1 onion
3 bay leaves, dried
6 cloves garlic
1 large chicken (about 4.4 lbs or 2 kg)
bunch fresh parsley
bunch fresh thyme
1 tbsp (15 ml) sea salt
pepper
about 12.5 cups (3 liters) water

CHICKEN SOUP

Peel the vegetables and cut into large pieces.

The chicken should be washed inside and outside with cold water.

Place a large stockpot on the stove. Put the veggies on the bottom of the pot, then on top of the veggies add the chicken and sprinkle with sea salt and pepper. Add two-thirds of the herbs.

Fill with water until the whole chicken is covered.

Simmer the soup just below the boiling point for 2–2.5 hours.

From time to time, skim the foam so that a clear chicken broth is created.

Remove the chicken and cut into pieces. Also remove the vegetables.

Pour the broth through a sieve into a smaller pot and let it boil for 5–10 minutes.

Season with salt and pepper and add the remaining fresh, chopped herbs.

SERVING SUGGESTIONS

Set aside approximately 4.2 oz (120 g) chicken meat and part of the vegetables in a soup bowl. Fill with the broth and garnish with herbs.

Serve the chicken on Caesar Salad (recipe page 176).

Serve the chicken with Nut Pesto (recipe page 110) and roasted vegetables or vegetable noodles.

3–4 SERVINGS

12 chicken wings, with skin
1 packet (0.4 oz or 12 g) of baking powder (gluten-free)
1 tsp (5 ml) sea salt
1 tbsp (15 ml) paprika or curry powder (optional)

CRISPY CHICKEN WINGS

PREPARATION

Preheat the oven to 250°F (120°C). Put a baking tray on the bottom of the oven to collect the dripping fat.

Wash the chicken wings and pat dry with paper towels. Mix baking powder and salt and evenly sprinkle on the chicken wings.

Place the wings onto a rack and roast so that the fat can drip down. Slide this into the lower third of the oven and bake for 30 minutes.

Place the rack a little higher in the oven and increase the heat to 425°F (220°C). Bake the wings for another 30–45 minutes.

SERVING SUGGESTIONS

Serve with a large green salad and Tomato Mayonnaise.

CHICKEN LIVER PÂTÉ

1 small onion
2 cloves garlic
3.5 oz (100 g) chestnut mushrooms
1.7 oz (50 g) butter
10.5 oz (300 g) chicken livers
   (tendons removed, ready to cook, 200 g)
1 pinch ground cloves
2 tbsp (30 ml) dry sherry or brandy (optional)
salt
pepper

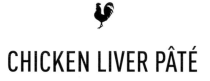

CHICKEN LIVER PÂTÉ

PREPARATION

Finely chop onion and garlic. Rinse the chicken livers in cold water,
drain in a colander, remove the tendons, and cut into small pieces.
Clean the mushrooms and cut them into quarters.

Melt the butter in a frying pan (at most medium heat).
Fry onion and garlic until soft, around 10 to 15 minutes.

Add the liver and mushrooms to the pan and cook for a further 10 minutes.

Pour the entire contents of the frying pan into a mixing bowl and puree
with a hand blender or in a food processor.
Add sherry or brandy and season with salt and pepper.

Put the pâté into a sealable container and place in the refrigerator
for at least 4 hours.

SERVING SUGGESTIONS

Serve with popovers (recipe page 120).

Serve with raw vegetables (e.g., celery, endive),
stuffed in hollowed cherry tomatoes, or spread on cucumber slices.

Serve on steamed or fried vegetable slices
(e.g., beets, sweet potatoes, pumpkin).

6–8 SERVINGS

1 organic grilled chicken
1 tbsp sea salt
black pepper or cayenne pepper
  (very hot) ground
6 fresh rosemary stalks
approximately 10.5 oz (300 g) potatoes
  or sweet potatoes and various other seasonal
  vegetables, prepared and cut into large pieces
salt
pepper

BUTTERFLY CHICKEN

Preheat the oven heat to 350°F (180°C). Line a tray with baking paper.
Wash the chicken inside and out with cold water.
Pat dry inside and out with paper towel.

With a knife or kitchen scissors, cut out the backbone
along the spine of the chicken.

Sprinkle salt and pepper generously over the chicken,
with its belly flat down on a baking sheet.

Slide the rosemary stalks gently under the skin. Again sprinkle some salt
on the skin and place in the oven for a total of 1 hour.

After 30 minutes, remove the baking sheet, add the potatoes and vegetables,
and coat them with the chicken fat. Add salt and pepper and bake for
another 30 minutes.

If after 1 hour the skin isn't crispy enough, you can turn on the broiler
and crisp the chicken for 5 minutes.

SERVING SUGGESTIONS

Divide the chicken into portions, one portion of approximately 2.1 oz (60 g) from
the bright, lean meat (breast) and 2.1 oz (60 g) of dark, fattier meat (wing, leg),
including skin, on each plate and serve with vegetables and potatoes.

Leftovers can be refrigerated three to four days.

DUCK BREAST OR QUAIL

PREPARATION

Wash the fillets/breasts with cold water and pat dry.

With a sharp knife, cut the skin crosswise (about 0.1–0.2 in or 3–5 mm deep, down to but not into the meat).

Season the fillets all over with salt and pepper.

Heat a frying pan on medium heat and put the duck breast fillets/quail with skin side down in the pan. As soon as the fat from the skin of the duck breast begins to melt into the pan, place the rosemary in the pan.
Fry until the skin is golden brown and crispy.
If necessary, from time to time drain the grease, so that the skin isn't floating in the fat.

Once the skin is golden brown and crispy, turn fillets/breasts and finish frying on the flesh side. Cooking to medium rare takes about 20 minutes together on both sides.

Remove from heat and let stand 5–10 minutes before slicing.

SERVING SUGGESTIONS

Cut the duck breast fillets/quail crosswise into strips
and serve with root puree (recipe page 96) and fruit sauce
(e.g., plum compote, apple sauce, or cranberry sauce).

Baked peaches go wonderfully with this recipe.

Serve cold with Caesar Salad (recipe page 176).

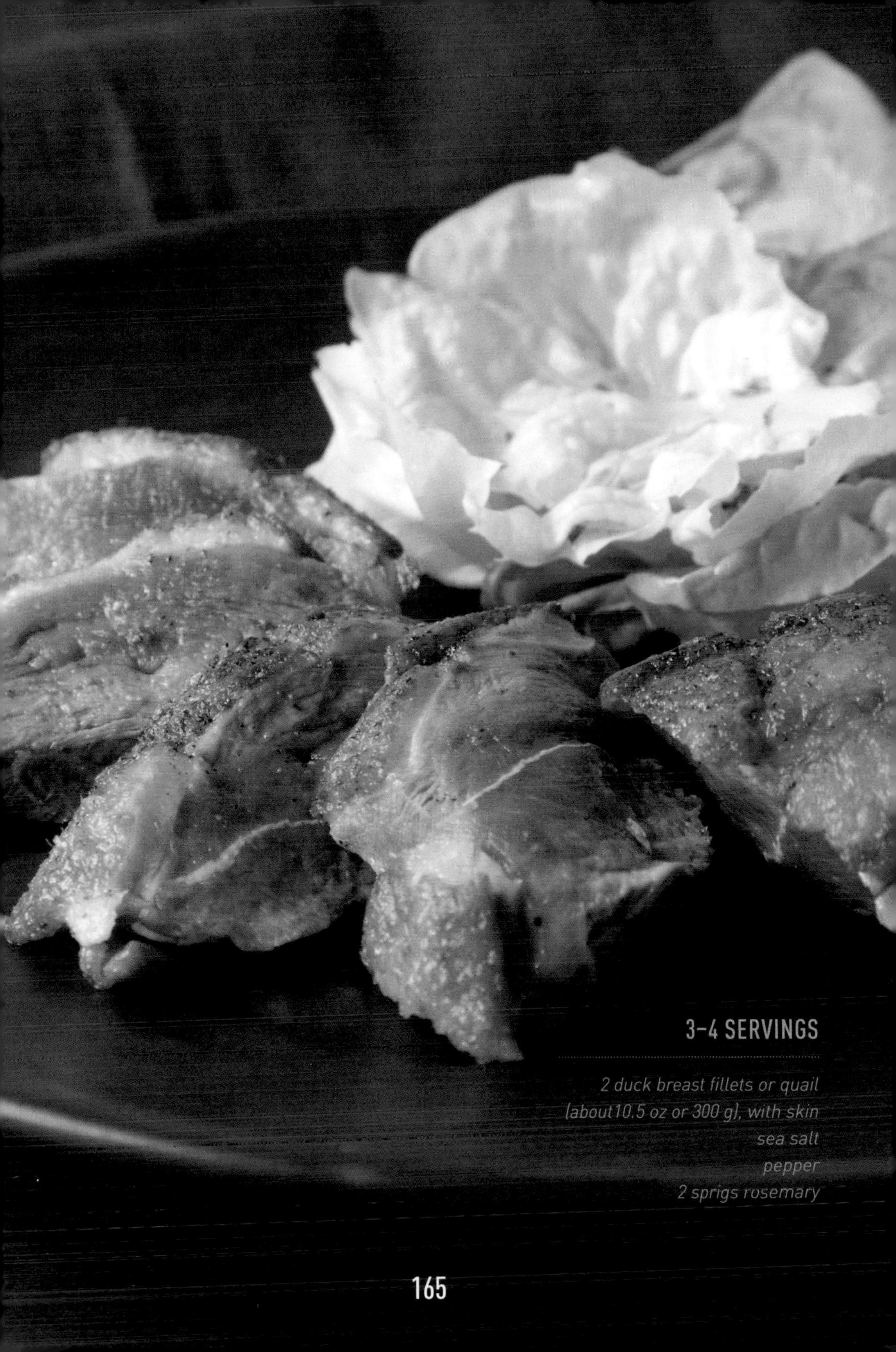

3–4 SERVINGS

2 duck breast fillets or quail (about10.5 oz or 300 g), with skin
sea salt
pepper
2 sprigs rosemary

FISH OIL

OMEGA-3 FATTY ACID LEVELS OF DIFFERENT FISH

The omega-3 fatty acids docosahexaenoic acid (DHA) and eicosapentaenoic acid (EPA) are found in fish.

- Wild-caught salmon, raw, cooked, or smoked: 1.8 percent
- Anchovies in olive oil: 1.7 percent
- Sardines, cooked, marinated in tomato sauce, or conserved in salt (preferably eaten with bones): 1.4 percent
- Atlantic herring, pickled: 1.2 percent
- Atlantic mackerel, cooked or smoked: 1 percent
- Tuna in olive oil, water, or salt: 0.7 percent

HIGH CONTENT OF OMEGA-3 FAT IN VEGETABLE OILS

Vegetable oils, for example linseed oil, chia seeds, and rapeseed oil, have far higher levels of omega-3 than fish. These are almost exclusively the omega-3 fatty acid alpha-linolenic acid. Unfortunately, humans can absorb and use only about 5 percent of these. As such, the smaller amounts of omega-3 found in fish are much more effective for humans.

ARE FISH OIL SUPPLEMENTS (E.G., FISH OIL CAPSULES) A GOOD ALTERNATIVE?

We'd do better to reduce our omega-6 consumption rather than supplement-ing with omega-3. Fish oil is a processed oil, like seed oils. It contains many polyunsaturated fatty acids, which are very unstable and oxidate easily, unlike natural, monounsaturated fatty acids (e.g., fatty acids in avocados or olive oil) and saturated fat. Omega-3s from real food (fish and seafood) are better pro-tected from oxidation.

The preparation of fish oil is comparable to that of vegetable oil. It is heated and treated with chemical agents so that the taste is tolerable and the oil is edible. It may well be, therefore, that well-intentioned supplementation with fish oil is in fact detrimental. Industrially produced, polyunsaturated omega-3 fatty acids aggravate chronic inflammation, rather than curing it.

FISH OIL FATTY ACID PROFILE

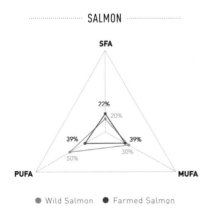

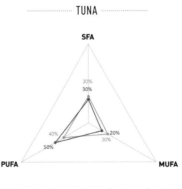

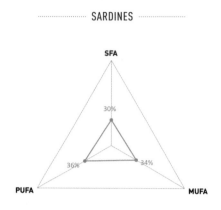

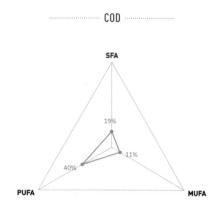

SFA = saturated fatty acids
PUFA = polyunsaturated fatty acids
MUFA = monounsaturated fatty acids

RECIPES

In these recipes we use only organic fish from sustainable farms or sustainably caught wild fish.

Conventionally farmed fish are kept in a small space and fattened unnaturally. If we want healthy polyunsaturated fatty acid, omega-3 fatty acid, we can't compromise on the quality of the fish we eat.

Canned fish (tuna, sardines, and anchovies) must be packaged in olive oil or salt water—not sunflower and/or soybean oil.

Most recipes can be prepared with different types of fish. If you don't want to eat raw fish, replace it with cooked or canned.

Smaller fish such as sardines have the advantage of being less polluted. Also, you can often eat the entire small fish, including bones, and therefore take in many more minerals and vitamins. Use fresh or frozen fish. When buying unwrapped fish, you have to make sure that it is freshly caught.

FEATURES OF FRESH FISH

WHOLE FISH		FRESH	OLD
Odor		light, pleasantly reminiscent of algae	sour smell of ammonia
Appearance	Skin	strong, shiny color, watery clear mucus	soft, dull color, matte mucus coating
	Eyes	plump, glossy, black, bright pupil	sunken, dull, milky gray pupil
	Gills	vibrant color, wet, shiny without mucus	brownish, yellowish, dry milky mucus
FILLET		firm and elastic, smooth surface, shimmering	limp, rough surface, dull, mottled

FISH: PREPARATION AND PROCESSING

Before preparing any kind of fish, always **wash**, **acidify**, and **salt**

Wash: You must remove the organs, scales, and fins from fish you're going to cook whole. Fresh fish, whether whole or already cut, are then thoroughly rinsed under running water. Fresh fish should not be soaked; this will make it lose valuable nutrients.

Acidify: The cleaned fish meat is drizzled on both sides with lemon juice. The acid removes the fishy smell and flavors the meat at the same time. In addition, the acid strengthens the structure of the meat and brightens it up a bit.

Salt: The fish is sprinkled with a little salt last. Salt pulls water out of the fish, which is why you only salt it just before cooking.

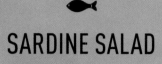

SARDINE SALAD

PREPARATION

Cut cucumber and beets into slices.

Arrange lettuce, cucumber, and beets on a plate. Sprinkle with salt and pepper.

Open the can of sardines and let the oil trickle over the salad (if the oil in the
can is not extra-virgin olive oil, then discard and substitute with high-quality oil).
Place the sardines whole or crushed on the salad and sprinkle
with finely chopped chives.

1 SERVING

1 can of sardines in extra-virgin olive oil (3.1 oz or 90 g)
1.7 oz (50 g) lettuce, washed and spun dry
3.5 oz (100 g) cucumber, peeled
3.5 oz (100 g) beetroot, cooked and peeled
fresh chives, washed
salt
pepper
spring onions (optional)

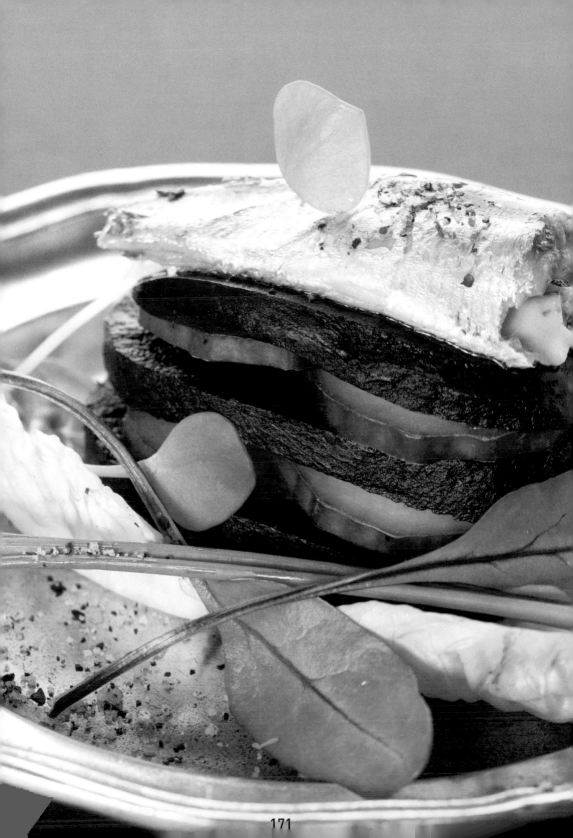

3–4 SERVINGS

4 whole trout, ready to cook (no organs, fins, etc.)
2 lemons, washed and cut into 8 slices
1 bunch fresh cilantro, washed
1.5 inches (4 cm) fresh ginger, peeled, thinly sliced
1 tbsp (15 ml) olive oil
sea salt
pepper

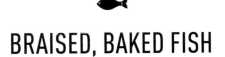

BRAISED, BAKED FISH

PREPARATION

Preheat the oven heat to 350°F (180°C).

Prepare 4 pieces of aluminum foil
(each about 31–39 inches or 80–100 cm long).

Wash the fish in cold water. Dry gently with paper towels.

Rub the fish well inside and outside with salt and pepper, and stuff the belly
of each fish with two slices of lemon, fresh ginger, and herbs
(divide ginger and herbs equally between the fish).

Sprinkle the aluminum foil with olive oil and put a stuffed trout on each piece.

Wrap the fish with aluminum foil and seal the edges well.

Place all aluminum fish packets on a baking sheet
and bake 20–25 minutes in the oven.

SERVING SUGGESTIONS

Take the fish carefully from the foil and put each on a big plate.
Serve with lettuce, vegetables, and/or root puree (recipe page 96).

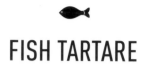

FISH TARTARE

PREPARATION

Cut the fish fillet into small pieces.

In a bowl, combine the tamari sauce with a little wasabi paste mix.
Gently stir in the fish pieces and marinate in the refrigerator for 10 minutes.

Cut the avocado into small pieces.

SERVING SUGGESTIONS

Serve with ring mold:
Place the ring on the plate.

Fill the ring with cooked rice and press it down. Place the avocado on top of the rice,
and also press it down. Place the fish on top of the avocado.

Remove the ring and garnish with spring onions, chives, and mayonnaise.
If you don't have a ring mold, line a small bowl with plastic wrap.
Layer in first the fish, then the avocado, and then the rice. Press lightly on the rice.
Put a plate on top of the bowl and turn the whole thing upside down.
Carefully lift up the bowl and remove the plastic wrap if it has clung to the food.
Garnish with spring onions, chives, and mayonnaise.

ALTERNATIVES

Instead of using raw fish, try fried or poached.
Strained fish (pickled in salt water) from a can also works well.

Instead of wasabi mayonnaise, you could use wasabi guacamole (recipe page 56–57).
The mayonnaise is optional.

Low-carb version: Create the tartare with cauliflower rice.

TIP

Cauliflower Rice—a low-carbohydrate rice substitute
Prepare, wash, and chop a cauliflower in a food processor.
The cauliflower pieces should be about the size of rice grains.
Cauliflower Rice can be cooked briefly in clarified butter, blanched in salted water
for 2–3 minutes, or microwaved until tender.

1 SERVING

3.5 oz (100 g) fresh salmon or tuna fillet
1 tbsp (15 ml) tamari sauce (gluten-free)
wasabi paste (quantity to taste, very spicy/gluten-free)
1.7 oz (50 g) avocado, peeled
3.5 oz (100 g) sushi rice or risotto rice, cooked (hot or cold)
chives and spring onions, cut into thin rings (optional)
wasabi mayonnaise (optional, recipe page 198)

3–4 SERVINGS

14.1 oz (400 g) sweet potatoes
1–2 tbsp (15–30 ml) butter, melted
4 anchovy fillets in olive oil, drained
1 clove garlic, peeled and finely chopped
3 tbsp (45 ml) olive oil
2 egg yolks (or 2 tbsp or 30 ml mayonnaise with olive oil)
lemon juice to taste
0.9 oz (25 g) freshly, finely grated Parmesan
1.7 oz (50 g) freshly shaved Parmesan
salt
pepper
2 heads romaine lettuce,
  washed, spun dry, and cut into large pieces
0.9–1.1 lbs (400–500 g) chicken or duck breast,
  roasted, or boiled shrimp, or salmon fillet

CAESAR SALAD WITH
SWEET POTATO CROUTONS

PREPARATION

Line a tray with baking paper. Turn the broiler on to medium.
Place the empty baking tray in the oven.

Peel and cut the sweet potatoes into equal-sized cubes (about 0.4 in or 1 cm).

Take the hot baking tray from the oven and melt butter on it. Add the sweet potato cubes
on the sheet and coat with the melted butter. Salt the sweet potatoes and return the tray
to the oven for 10–20 minutes.

Halfway through, rotate the cubes. Once they are brown and crispy, remove from the oven.

For the dressing, crush the anchovies and the garlic clove in a mortar to form a paste.
Place in a large salad bowl and mix well with olive oil, egg yolks, lemon juice, and grated
Parmesan. If the sauce needs more liquid, add water until it has the right consistency.

SERVING SUGGESTIONS

Place the romaine lettuce on a plate, then sprinkle with shaved Parmesan
and sweet potato croutons. Spread the dressing over the chicken strips
(or the cooked prawns or poached salmon) and place on the plate too.

3-4 SERVINGS

10.5 oz (300 g) beetroot
10.5 oz (300 g) sweet potatoes
10.5 oz (300 g) parsnips or parsley root
1 tbsp (15 ml) coconut oil, liquid
salt
pepper
1.8 lb (800 g) fish fillet
(e.g., perch, cod, trout, salmon)
1 tbsp (15 ml) coconut oil
salt
pepper
4 portions mayonnaise (recipe page 198)

FISH AND VEGETABLE STICKS

PREPARATION

Preheat the oven to 350°F (180°C), line a baking sheet with parchment paper,
and place in the oven to warm up.

Cut the beetroot, sweet potatoes, and parsnips into equal-sized fries.

Remove the baking sheet from the oven, spread the coconut oil on it,
and place the vegetables in layers with salt and pepper.
Return to the oven for 20 minutes, turning after 10 minutes.

Preheat the broiler and broil the fries for about 10 to 20 minutes until they are crispy.

While the vegetables are roasting, wash the fish fillets and pat dry, then season with
salt and pepper on both sides.

In a frying pan warm 1 tbsp of coconut oil on medium heat, then fry the fillets about
2–4 minutes each side, depending on the type of fish.

SERVING SUGGESTIONS

Place the different colored vegetable sticks on a plate next to the fish fillets
and put the mayonnaise in a small bowl.

MILK FAT

The fat in cow's milk is very complex, consisting of 95 percent triglycerides. These triglycerides contain more than 60 different fatty acids. There is a relatively high content of medium and short chain fatty acids.

The proportion of unsaturated fatty acids varies and depends on the season, the type of feeding, and the breed. Highland cattle supplies, for example, less but fattier milk, while Netherlands cattle create more milk that has much less fat. Cheese, butter, clarified butter, yogurt, cottage cheese, and many other products are manufactured from milk. These all include different levels of milk fat too. To be able to obtain optimum nutrients (fatty acids, vitamins, etc.) from the milk, it must not be pasteurized or homogenized.

All pasteurized and homogenized milk products are denatured, and thus become unrecognizable to the body, generating problems in digestion and metabolization— for example, digestive upset, headaches, obesity, a runny nose, and much more. The retail sale of raw milk is not legal in all states; in some you may have to go to the farm to buy it, or participate in a herd share.

In a few states, all sales are outright illegal. Do your best to find the highest-quality dairy you can.

Just as important as the natural structure of the food is its quality. Milk from cows that are fed on GM crops is not a healthy food in its raw state. Because of the grains the cows eat, the milk's fatty acid structure changes and contains more omega-6 than that of cows that are not fed grains. If you consume milk and dairy products, then source it from cows fed on pasture grass in the summer and hay in the winter. Cows raised and fed in a species-appropriate manner provide foods that are full of nutrients, meaning we can eat smaller portions yet ingest far more vitamins, fatty acids, and minerals than we can from milk and milk products from conventionally reared and fattened animals.

High-quality dairy products are more expensive, but they're worth the price for me, because of the welfare of the animal and because of my own health. I'm also saving money for myself and my company— I take far fewer sick days and have lower medical and drug costs because I'm willing to invest in the food I buy.

RAW-MILK BUTTER MORE HEALTHY THAN PREVIOUSLY THOUGHT

Myristic acid, a saturated fatty acid found in the natural form of raw-milk butter, has a favorable effect on the fat and cholesterol in the blood and on the ratio between the "good" (HDL) and "bad" (LDL) cholesterols.

Raw-milk butter also contains the vital substance cholesterol. The body needs cholesterol to form, for example, cortisone (important for circadian rhythm), sex hormones, vitamin D, and bile acid. Cholesterol (from raw-milk butter, eggs, etc.) is therefore essential for our health. The fear of too much cholesterol in the diet is unfounded, because the "external" supply of cholesterol affects blood cholesterol levels to only 10–20 percent. Anyone with a lower proportion who eats according to the Pure Food principles need hardly be worried about their cholesterol levels, because this diet promotes health via many different mechanisms in the body.

HIGHEST QUALITY BUTTER

Most butter is pasteurized to make it last longer. Unfortunately, only raw-milk butter can ensure that the fatty acids (also myristic acid and cholesterol, as well as the entire nutritional composition) remain absolutely unchanged, so that the body can easily recognize, absorb, and metabolize them.

The best raw-milk butter is produced from the milk of pastured horned cows eating mainly fresh grass and herbs, because their raw milk contains a good amount of omega-3 fatty acids.

It's hard to find raw-milk butter, but it's worth it if you can get it.

MILK FAT FATTY ACID PROFILE

BUTTER

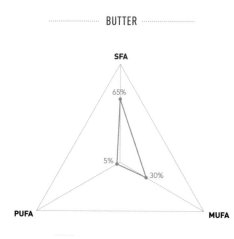

CLARIFIED BUTTER

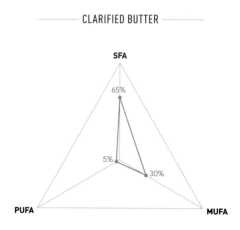

SFA = saturated fatty acids
PUFA = polyunsaturated fatty acids
MUFA = monounsaturated fatty acids

RECIPES

I use only raw milk and raw-milk products. Again, these can be hard to find in the United Sates—often your best bet will be to buy directly from a farm. It's important to source raw dairy whenever you can.

Clarified butter can be heated up to 350°F (180°C). It is ideal for frying meat, fish, eggs, poultry, and vegetables. Clarified butter is created by heating butter until the melted butter fat separates from the water and protein components. The water and protein are skimmed off, and the melted butter is bottled and sold as cooking butter. The clarified butter contains a water content of just 0.2 percent (butter contains about 16 percent water). Clarified butter can be kept chilled and is more durable than butter. Ghee is the common cooking butter in Indian and Pakistani cuisine. It also has a long tradition in Ayurvedic cooking.

Clarified butter/ghee gives food a nutty flavor and makes, for example, hash browns crispy. In all recipes butter or clarified butter can be replaced by coconut oil, depending on your taste preference.

There are three fat levels of raw-milk cheese: full-fat, semi-fat, and skim. In the recipes I consciously provide a fat level to make a well-balanced recipe as a whole. In the Muesli with Raw Milk (recipe page 105), I use low-fat raw-milk quark because the muesli already contains a lot of fat; the quark is providing the protein instead.

If you're following a ketogenic diet, you cannot eat medium or low-fat milk products because they contain too many carbs and proteins.

SPICED BUTTER ROLLS

PREPARATION

Mix room-temperature butter with the finely chopped ingredients.

Pour the spiced butter on a transparent sheet and form into a roll. Solidify in the refrigerator or freezer. You can also put the butter in a small bowl or glass.

SERVING SUGGESTIONS

Spiced butter goes well with steamed vegetables and seared lean meats, poultry, and fish.

CHIVE BUTTER

4.4 oz (125 g) butter
1.7 oz (50 g) fresh chives
½ lemon (juice and peel),
 peel finely grated
naturally flavored salt
 with lemon peel, or sea salt
pepper

ANCHOVY BUTTER

4.4 oz (125 g) butter
5 anchovy fillets, pickled in brine, drained
black pepper, freshly ground

ITALIAN HERB BUTTER

4.4 oz (125 g) butter
1.7 oz (50 g) herbs
  (e.g., basil, oregano, thyme, parsley)
1 clove garlic
salt
pepper

TOMATO BUTTER

4.4 oz (125 g) butter
1.7 oz (50 g) tomato paste
1 tsp (5 ml) pepper
sea salt

RÖSTI WITH FRIED EGG

PREPARATION

In a bowl place the grated sweet potatoes with egg whites, coconut flour, and salt and mix well.

In a large nonstick skillet, heat 2 tbsp (30 ml) clarified butter on medium-high. If you want to add onion and/or fried bacon, fry them in the clarified butter until soft.

Spread the potatoes evenly over the onions and press down slightly.

Reduce the heat to medium, cover the pan, and cook for about 10 minutes.

Place a large, shallow dish on the potatoes and turn the pan over. Now the already fried side of the rösti is on top of the plate.

Pour the remaining clarified butter into the pan and let the hash browns slide off the plate onto the pan. Fry again for 5–10 minutes.

In a separate pan, fry the eggs.

SERVING SUGGESTIONS

Instead of a big rösti, divide the grated potatoes into three or four servings. Goes well with Oriental Lamb Stew (recipe page 150) or Butter Chicken (recipe page 188).

3-4 SERVINGS

1.8 lb (800 g) sweet potatoes,
peeled and coarsely grated
4 egg whites
2 tbsp (30 m) coconut flour
1 tsp (5 ml) salt
pepper
1 onion, peeled and chopped (optional)
3.5 oz (100 g) fried bacon, cut into cubes or strips
(optional)
4 tbsp (60 ml) clarified butter
4 eggs
1 tbsp (15 ml) clarified butter
salt
pepper

187

3–4 SERVINGS

1.3 lbs (600 g) chicken breast
2 tbsp (30 ml) clarified butter
2 tbsp (30 ml) butter
2 tsp (10 ml) garam masala (optional)
2 tsp (10 ml) paprika ground
2 tsp (10 ml) ground coriander
1 tbsp (15 ml) fresh ginger or 1 tsp (5 ml) crushed ginger
1 tsp (5 ml) chili flakes
1 stick of cinnamon, dried or 1 tsp (5 ml) cinnamon, ground
1 tsp (5 ml) ground turmeric
1 can tomato puree
approximately 0.4 cup (100 ml) cream (not homogenized!)
1 tbsp (15 ml) lemon juice
sea salt
1 tsp (5 ml) raw sugar (optional)

BUTTER CHICKEN

PREPARATION

Cut the chicken breasts into pieces.

In a large skillet heat the clarified butter and fry the chicken.
Set the chicken aside.

In the same pan, melt 2 tbsp (30 ml) butter over medium heat
and sauté all the spices in it.

As soon as a thick, fragrant paste is formed, add the tomato puree and boil.
Reduce the heat and add cream. Add some lemon juice, salt, and a little sugar.
Don't boil the sauce. Add the fried chicken and cook until just warm.

SERVING SUGGESTIONS

Serve with cauliflower rice (recipe page 175) or boiled rice.

1 SWEET MEAL OR
2–3 DESSERTS | PAVLOVA

1 egg white
0.4 oz (10 g) icing sugar
0.2 oz (5 g) cocoa powder (unsweetened)
0.4 oz (10 g) almonds, ground

COCOA QUARK CREAM

2 egg whites
0.7 oz (20 g) icing sugar
0.4 oz (10 g) cocoa powder
3.5 oz (100 g) raw-milk quark, skim
3.5 oz (100 g) raw-milk quark, full fat
1.7 oz (50 g) berries

CHOCOLATE PAVLOVA WITH COCOA QUARK CREAM

PREPARATION PAVLOVA

Preheat the oven to 320°F (160°C). Line a tray with baking paper.
Beat 1 egg white until stiff, sprinkle in the icing sugar, and continue to mix.
Sift the cocoa powder over the egg whites and mix together gently.
Carefully fold in the ground almonds.

Draw 6 circles with a 1.6 in (4 cm) diameter on the baking paper,
then spread the pavlova in the circles.

Bake 30 minutes in the lower third of the oven.

Cool entirely on the baking paper.

PREPARATION COCOA QUARK CREAM

In a bowl, beat the egg whites until stiff.
In a second bowl mix skim- and whole-milk quark. Sift the cocoa powder and
icing sugar over the quark and blend well. Carefully fold the stiff egg whites
into the chocolate quark mix.

SERVING SUGGESTIONS

Simple version:
Pour cream into bowls and garnish with berries and pavlova.

Elegant version:
The pavlova pile (picture).

191

BUTTER COFFEE 1 CUP

1 cup coffee, freshly brewed
2 tbsp (30 ml) butter (if possible from raw milk)
1 pinch cinnamon

COCONUT COFFEE 1 CUP

1 cup freshly brewed coffee
2 tbsp (30 ml) virgin coconut oil
1 pinch cinnamon

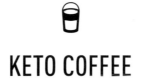

KETO COFFEE

Pour the coffee into a mixing bowl, then add the butter/coconut oil and cinnamon. With a hand blender or food processor, mix vigorously until some foam has formed and the fat/oil has mixed with the coffee.

TIP

In order to not break your fast and to keep metabolizing fat for energy, drink a coffee with butter or coconut oil.

The Keto Coffee gives you a mental kick via the caffeine and some more energy from the butter/coconut oil.

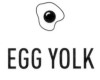

EGG YOLK

The color of an eggshell is genetically determined and depends on the breed of hen that laid it. Purebred chickens with white earlobes almost always lay eggs with white shells, while chickens with red earlobes usually lay eggs with brown shells.
The color of the eggshell does not affect the nutritional content of the egg. The care and feeding of the animals, however, have a major impact on the nutrients.

In mass production, hybrid chickens are used, optimized to produce more than 300 eggs per year. To breed chickens, all eggs are hatched, but roosters are of no use to the egg industry; therefore, they are gassed with CO_2 or shredded. Worldwide, 2.5 billion roosters die due to this practice.

The life of these animals in factory farming is bleak—constant stress and a fight for space and food. The animals are kept healthy with medication and fattened with grain, with the sole aim of regular egg production.

Such eggs not only contain fewer nutrients—they're directly harmful. Firstly, they are energetically negatively charged due to the stressed animal. Secondly, such eggs contain lots of anti-nutrients from the chickens' unnatural grain diet, and the residue of antibiotics given to the chickens. The fatty acid profile is also different in factory-farmed eggs, with much more omega-6 than in eggs from naturally raised chickens.

Eggs from hens that are allowed to find their natural food outdoors and don't have to lay an egg every day contain many healthy nutrients that can easily be absorbed and used in the human body. This includes lecithin, which is important to brain function, and also lutein and zeaxanthin, important for the function of the retina. Last but not least, eggs from hens that are kept free and permitted to eat humanely have a significantly higher omega-3 fatty acid content.

The ideal storage in the household is in the refrigerator at 41°F–53°F (5°C–12°C). Warm temperatures are bad for the freshness of the egg.

For dishes in which the egg is not heated (such as cold sauces), always use very fresh eggs.

EGG YOLK FATTY ACID PROFILE

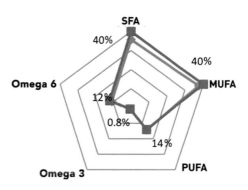

—◆— whole egg

—■— egg yolk

SFA = saturated fatty acids
PUFA = polyunsaturated fatty acids
MUFA = monounsaturated fatty acids

RECIPE

In these recipes I always use organic eggs from the supermarket or eggs directly from the farmer. I like to go to the farms, where I can see how the animals are raised and fed. I can ask the farmer all my questions and buy the eggs much cheaper than in a supermarket! The eggs are usually small (1.9 oz, or 55 g) to large (2.1 oz, or 60 g).

SHELF LIFE

Eggs with undamaged shells are shelf stable and fresh for at least three weeks after being laid. If they're kept in the fridge, they're usually fine for up to five weeks.

A fresh, whole egg has a natural protection that prevents germs from multiplying in the egg for up to three weeks after laying.

FRESH TEST

The porous eggshell lets the liquid inside evaporate during prolonged storage. To the same extent as the liquid evaporates, the air bubble in the egg grows. With this floating test you can determine the freshness of eggs. A fresh egg has a small air bubble and is heavier than water; it will sink in a glass of water. As the air bubble gets larger, the egg will stand on its end; a three-week-old egg will float up to the surface of the water and is past eating.

195

1 SERVING
....

2 raw eggs
3.5 oz (100 g) banana
3.5 oz (100 g) spinach leaves, washed
avocado
1 tsp vanilla powder
1 tsp turmeric, ground
0.4–0.8 cups (100–200 ml) water or ice cubes (optional)

SMOOTHIE WITH EGG

Put all ingredients in a mixing bowl and blend finely
with a hand blender or in a food processor.

WASABI MAYONNAISE

Mix 1–2 tsp (5-10 ml) wasabi paste with the finished basic mayonnaise.

HERB MAYONNAISE

Mix bunch of fresh, finely chopped herbs with the finished basic mayonnaise.

TOMATO MAYONNAISE

Mix 1–2 tbsp (15–30 ml) tomato puree with the finished basic mayonnaise.

MAYONNAISE VARIATIONS

PREPARATION

Find a jar that can hold 1 cup (250 ml) of liquid and ensure your hand blender can be inserted through the opening down to the glass bottom.

Pour the olive oil and all the other ingredients into the jar.

Keep the hand blender in the jar, so that it reaches all the way to the bottom. Mix for 1 minute without moving the hand blender.

Move the hand blender slowly up about an inch (3–4 cm) and then move back down slowly. Repeat this three times.

Taste the mayonnaise and, if necessary, add a little salt.

SHELF LIFE

It will keep in a mason jar in the refrigerator for one week.

SERVING SUGGESTIONS

Mayonnaise goes very well with fish fillets, vegetables, and potato or Coconut Sweet Potato Chips (recipe page 78).

You can make a quick meal with a can of tuna (stored in salt water), a helping of mayonnaise, and a crisp green salad.

BASIC OLIVE OIL MAYONNAISE

0.8 cups (200 ml) olive oil (choose very mild oil,
  so that the mayonnaise is not bitter)
1 egg
1 tsp (5 ml) mustard or mustard powder
a little lemon juice, freshly squeezed
sea salt, optional

SWEET POTATO-SHRIMP SALAD

PREPARATION

Peel the sweet potatoes and cut into small cubes.

In a saucepan, boil water, add salt, and cook the sweet potatoes until soft (about 15 minutes). Allow to cool slightly.

Rinse the shrimp under cold water, pat dry with paper towel, and cut into small pieces. Cut the cherry tomatoes in half.

In a bowl, combine the shrimp, cherry tomatoes, sweet potatoes, and finely chopped herbs with the tomato mayonnaise. Season with salt and pepper.

ALTERNATIVES

Instead of using cooked shrimp, try chicken breast or boiled eggs.

3-4 SERVINGS

1.3 lbs (600 g) shrimp, cooked and peeled
5.6 oz (160 g) Tomato Mayonnaise (recipe page 198)
1 lb (480 g) sweet potatoes
7 oz (200 g) cherry tomatoes
salt
pepper
1 bunch fresh chives or cilantro

1 SERVING

2 eggs
1 egg yolk or 1 tbsp (15 ml) cream (optional)
salt
pepper
1 tbsp (15 ml) clarified butter
1 oz (30 g) Parmesan made
* from raw milk, freshly grated*
1 tomato, peeled and cut into small cubes

CHEESE OMELETTE

PREPARATION

Whisk the eggs in a bowl, add salt and pepper.

Heat a pan on medium with 1 tbsp (15 ml) clarified butter.

Pour the eggs into the pan. Let thicken for a few minutes.
Distribute the Parmesan and the diced tomatoes on the omelette while
the egg is still moist.

Fold the omelette and continue to fry another 2–3 minutes.
Then carefully slide the omelette onto a plate.

SERVING SUGGESTIONS

Serve with a portion of Coconut Sweet Potato Chips (recipe page 78).
Instead of incorporating diced tomatoes into the omelette,
you can also serve them separately.

VARIATIONS

Instead of Parmesan, use 1 oz (30 g) buffalo mozzarella, raw-milk feta, or Gruyère.

Instead of tomatoes, try steamed spinach, avocado, or guacamole (recipe page 56)
in the omelette.

EGGS AND VEGETABLE SALAD

PREPARATION

Wash the vegetables, then cut into pieces and cook until they're
just firm to the bite. Let cool.
In a bowl mix olive oil, lemon juice or vinegar, green onions, salt,
and pepper. Place the vegetables and the quartered eggs on plates,
pour the sauce, and sprinkle with the flaked almonds.

ALTERNATIVES

Instead of salad dressing for the sauce, use mayonnaise thinned with
a little water, broth, or olive oil.
Use other seasonal vegetables or root vegetables/potatoes.

3-4 SERVINGS

8.8 oz (250 g) broccoli
8.8 oz (250 g) cauliflower
7 oz (200 g) green asparagus
6 eggs, hard boiled, peeled and quartered
6-8 tbsp (90-120 ml) olive oil
1 tbsp (15 ml) lemon juice or vinegar
2 green onions, sliced into thin rings
sea salt or seasoned salt (e.g., orange or curry salt)
pepper
1.4 oz (40 g) flaked almonds, roasted

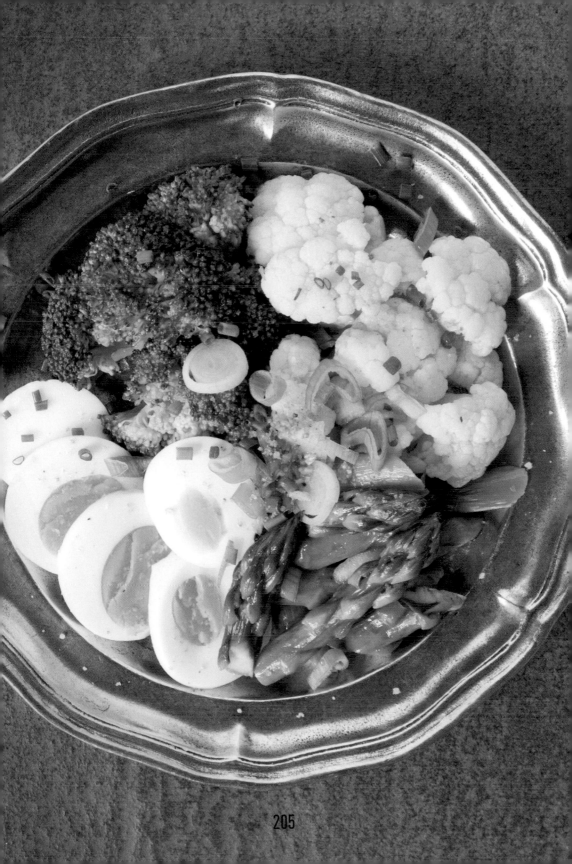

CHOCOLATE MOUSSE

PREPARATION

Separate the eggs and place in a bowl.

Whisk the egg whites with a pinch of salt until stiff.

Melt the chocolate in the microwave or in a double boiler. While you stir
the liquid chocolate constantly, mix in the egg yolks. Add a third of the stiff
egg whites to the chocolate-yolk mixture and blend well.

Mix the remaining stiff egg whites carefully by hand
into the chocolate mixture.

Divide between small glasses or bowls, cover with cling wrap, and place in
the refrigerator to set for at least 4 hours.

SERVING SUGGESTIONS

Put fresh berries or berry compote on the mousse.
Garnish with whipped heavy cream or whipped coconut cream
(recipe page 70–71).

4 eggs
3.5 oz (100 g) dark chocolate
(72 percent cocoa)
1 pinch of salt

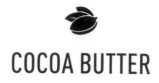

COCOA BUTTER

Last but not least: cocoa butter, one of my favorites. I don't use it for cooking and baking yet, but I regularly eat cocoa butter in dark chocolate. If you let a piece of dark chocolate (at least 70 percent cocoa) melt on your tongue, you can feel the soft, delicate texture of the cocoa butter. Chocolate should be at least 70 percent cocoa, so that the sugar content of the chocolate is not too high.

ABOUT COCOA BUTTER

Cocoa butter is the fat of the seeds of the cocoa plant, which is obtained by pressing the cocoa mass (so-called press butter) or by extraction with solvents (extraction butter). There is also expeller cocoa butter, which is obtained with screw presses from unpeeled cacao beans and shells.

There are different cocoa butter qualities available—organic, raw, and cold-pressed, or refined. You can buy cocoa butter in blocks, small pellets, or as a powder.

Cocoa butter has a specific consistency: below the melting range 89°F–97°F (32°C–36°C) it is hard and brittle and then suddenly begins to melt above those temperatures. This property is particularly important in the production of chocolate, giving it its ability to melt in the mouth—a characteristic so far not achieved by any replacement fat.

USES OF COCOA BUTTER

- In preparation of chocolate
- As a butter replacement in baked goods
- In smoothies
- For steaming vegetables and searing meat and fish
- As a skin cream or for hair care

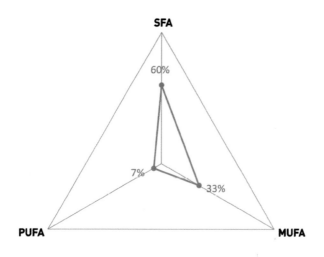

SFA = saturated fatty acids
PUFA = polyunsaturated fatty acids
MUFA = monounsaturated fatty acids

INGREDIENTS

INGREDIENTS

....

1.7 oz (50 g) cocoa butter
0.7 oz (20 g) sugar or honey
1 oz (30 g) cocoa powder
1 tsp (5 ml) vanilla powder

Optional toppings:
1 oz (30 g) nuts (whole or chopped)
0.7 oz (20 g) cocoa nibs (slightly bitter)
candied ginger
dried fruit (raisins, mango, apricot, etc.)
spices (cinnamon, coriander, sea salt, etc.)

PURE FOOD CHOCOLATE
(HOMEMADE CHOCOLATE)

PREPARATION

Melt cocoa butter in a bowl over water.
Once the cocoa butter is liquid, add the sugar or honey and stir until
the sugar has dissolved.

Add cocoa powder, vanilla powder, and/or spices and mix well.

The mass should still be slightly runny, so the chocolate can be
poured into small ramekins or in one large flat shape.
Before pouring, line whatever forms you use with plastic wrap so
that the chocolate can easily be removed after cooling. Then pour.

Spread any toppings you choose on top of the chocolate.
I like chocolate with a pinch of sea salt. Or in the winter,
with cinnamon and coriander.

Let harden in the refrigerator for at least 1 hour.

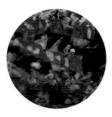
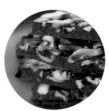
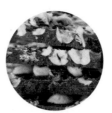
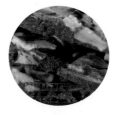

COCOA NIBS   PISTACHIO   HAZELNUT   DRIED MANGO

FINISHED?

The manuscript is finished! I'm happy and satisfied that I completed this huge amount of work in ten weeks without too much stress and illness.

While writing this book, I worked four days a week, worked out for a half hour every day, created and tested the recipes, and slept an average of seven hours a night. I ate three meals a day, two of which I cooked fresh. I wrote two outlines for new projects and spent time with my family. We went skiing almost every weekend during winter.

Where does the energy and joy come from for all these activities? I have nourished myself with a ketogenic diet for the last six weeks. I've been eating Pure Food for a few years. I don't eat grains, just more fat. On this ketogenic diet I have reduced my carbohydrates even further, eaten less protein, and increased my fat intake. This is actually the first time I've eaten ketogenically—normally I've followed the recommendations in my books over a lengthy period before writing, but not this time.

I adjusted my after-Christmas diet, and two days later, my head was clear. I could concentrate on my work for much longer periods. I was mentally agile and physically in top shape. I felt very aware that I was able to do more than before. I knew I had a lot of work in front of me and that I could do it. I was absolutely free from cravings for sugar and sweets. Sometimes in the evening, I looked at my carb calculator and realized I hadn't eaten all my allotted carbs. But despite eating a piece of chocolate, I was fine—and amazed at myself. How different I felt compared to my days as a carb addict, and even in comparison to my low-carb days.

I was, despite minimal carbohydrates in my diet (1 oz, or 30 g, or less daily), fit, and my strength-training performance was improving.

With my newly clear mind, I divided my time efficiently between all the important projects and tasks at hand. I made a detailed plan with bigger and smaller goals, steps, and milestones. I also planned my family time, spare time, and rest time. I never felt guilty about my family or myself.

I have a challenging job that includes taking care of a group of demanding clients who no one else can handle. Despite the bad news I have to convey, the discussions often turn into positive relationships. I believe I can manage these situations so well because I'm prepared, focused, and able to concentrate for longer periods. I'm calmer and self-confident enough to find a good answer or solution during each meeting.

I know I can't keep up such an intensive pace over longer periods, so even before I started to write this book, I planned a long family vacation for when the book was finished. It's tempting to be this efficient and effective all the time, but I'm convinced that it's not healthy over longer periods. The body will ask for a rest, and if we don't listen, we become sick. The time we then have to recover will be even longer. I've made a promise to myself not to let myself burn out like that.

There's so much left to say about fat and nutrition. I have so many more recipes I want to create and publish, and I could have worked on this manuscript for much longer. Then, a couple of days before it was due, I met Verena. She said, very convincingly, "You can write all that extra stuff in your next book." It helped me accept that a health guide can actually never be complete—there's so much new science and information discovered every day.

Verena, without realizing it, helped me to complete this book and have a relaxing family vacation.

Finished? Yes. For the moment.

ACKNOWLEDGMENTS

Thanks to my husband, Dave, and my son, Ray, for their patience and understanding when I did not always have time for them, and for trying all the recipes and suggesting improvements.

Thanks to Sibylla, who researched the history of fat phobia for me and wrote it down chronologically. She has helped to make this book easy to understand and interesting.

Thanks to Torsten, who with his medical knowledge easily describes the important scientific functions in the body. In addition, he checked my accumulated knowledge and my practical knowledge for correctness.

Thanks to Nadine, who calculated all the macronutrient contents for the meal plans, and asked all the annoying but necessary questions.

Thanks to Daniela and Benjamin for the beautiful photos. You transformed my ideas into wonderful pictures.

Thanks to the publisher for the freedom to create this book according to my ideas.

BIBLIOGRAPHY NOTE

In the original German edition of this book, the author included many excellent footnotes and bibliographical references. These can be found on her website, romydolle.com.

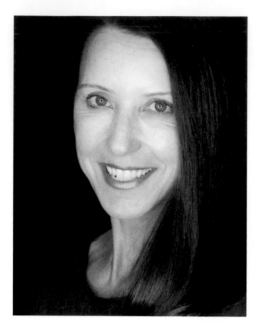

ROMY DOLLÉ

Romy is married to Dave Dollé and the mother of Ray (2005). She is a family woman and entrepreneur, she has an MBA in finance and has been working in the finance industry for more than twenty-five years, and she is an author.

Romy is curious and adventurous, willing to take risks and explore new areas in life. She is always eager to learn and develop mentally and physically. She loves to travel and explore new places, discover other cultures and foods. She cherishes family, friends and nature, and she's a strong believer that love and freedom go well together.

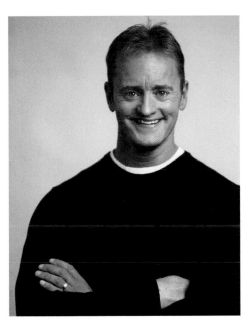

TORSTEN ALBERS, M.D.

Albers concepts, Zürich/Schlieren
www.albers-concepts.com

Torsten has a PhD in sports and nutrition. He is a former athlete and coach to professionals and amateur athletes. He gives advice in athletic training and nutrition, and also coaches entrepreneurs and executive managers to reduce stress and enhance performance and health.

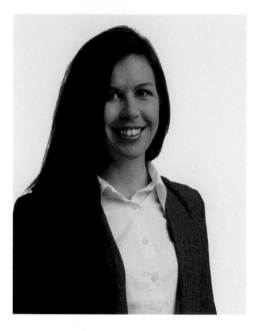

SIBYLLA ROTZLER

Sibylla is a journalist and corporate communications expert who lives and works in Zurich, Switzerland. She used to write articles for Dave Dollé's corporate blog about health, fitness, nutrition and other topics relevant to a modern healthy lifestyle.

One of her interests in life is the power of thought, and she enjoys exploring human behavior.

Sibylla was a great support in the research and writing of the history of fat for this book.

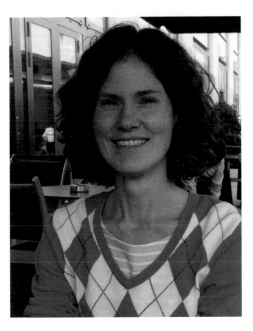

NADINE ESPOSITO

For as long as Nadine can remember, health and nutrition have been important topics in her life. She has studied the philosophy behind the primal lifestyle and Pure Food in depth. She is convinced that her healthy diet and happiness in life are balancing out her stressful job.

Nadine supported the team with all the macronutrient calculations and graphs.

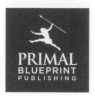

OTHER BOOKS BY
PRIMAL BLUEPRINT
PUBLISHING

MARK SISSON

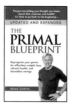

The Primal Connection: *Follow your genetic blueprint to health and happiness*

The Primal Blueprint: *Reprogram your genes for effortless weight loss, vibrant health, and boundless energy*

The Primal Blueprint 21-Day Total Body Transformation: *A step-by-step diet and lifestyle makeover to become a fat-burning machine!*

The Primal Blueprint 90-Day Journal: *A Personal Experiment (n=1)*

Primal Blueprint Box Set: *Includes the original "Primal Blueprint" hardcover, "The Primal Connection," "The Primal Blueprint Cookbook," "The Primal Blueprint Quick & Easy Meals," and "Primal Blueprint Healthy Sauces, Dressings & Toppings"*

MARK SISSON AND BRAD KEARNS

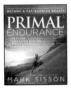 **Primal Endurance:** *Escape chronic cardio and carbohydrate dependency and become a fat-burning beast!*

COOKBOOKS BY MARK SISSON AND JENNIFER MEIER

 The Primal Blueprint Cookbook: *Primal, low carb, paleo, grain-free, dairy-free and gluten-free meals*

 The Primal Blueprint Quick and Easy Meals: *Delicous, Primal-approved meals you can make in under 30 minutes*

 The Primal Blueprint Healthy Sauces, Dressings, and Toppings: *Plus rubs, dips, marinades and other easy ways to transform basic natural foods into Primal masterpieces*

OTHER AUTHORS

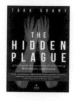

Hidden Plague: *A field guide for surviving and overcoming hidradenitis suppurativa,* by Tara Grant

Rich Food, Poor Food: *The Ultimate Grocery Purchasing System (GPS),* by Mira Calton, CN, and Jayson Calton, Ph.D.

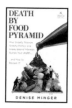

Death by Food Pyramid: *How shoddy science, sketchy politics and shady special interests ruined your health,* by Denise Minger

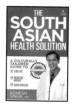

The South Asian Health Solution: *A culturally tailored guide to lose fat, increase energy, avoid disease,* by Ronesh Sinha, MD

Paleo Girl: *A straight talk guide to navigating the challenges of adolescence with a sensible, stress-balanced, Primal approach,* by Leslie Klenke

Lil' Grok Meets the Korgs: *A prehistoric boy shows a high tech modern family how to live Primally,* by Janée Meadows

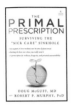 **The Primal Prescription:** *Suviving the "sick care" sinkhole,* by Doug McGuff, MD and Robert P. Murphy, PhD

COOKBOOKS

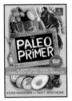 **The Paleo Primer:** *A jump-start guide to losing body fat and living Primally,* by Keris Marsden and Matt Whitmore

 Primal Cravings: *Your favorite foods made paleo,* by Brandon and Megan Keatley

 Fruit Belly: *A 4-day quick fix to relieve bloating caused by high carb, high fruit diets,* by Romy Dollé